INTERMITTENT FASTING FOR WOMEN OVER 60

INTERMITTENT FASTING FOR WOMEN OVER 60 YEARS TO LOSE WEIGHT, BURN FAT AND GET YOUR DESIRED SHAPE.

Table of contents

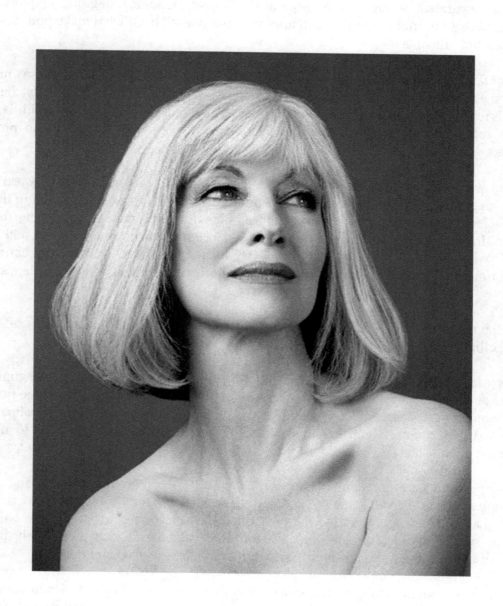

INTRODUCTION TO INTERMITTENT FASTING FOR WOMEN OVER 60

Many years of normal information have directed that the ideal approach to eat is to eat around six little meals separated a few hours separated. Notwithstanding, ongoing exploration has recommended that intermittent fasting can improve your overall health and make you less helpless against incessant ailments.

Intermittent fasting is a sustenance plan that can really fit into your life, and that doesn't make each and every meal an exercise in shuffling your calendar. While it isn't for everybody, individuals who are disappointed with their present dietary patterns might be keen on the health benefits of eating less regular meals and in a potential increment in your body's capacity to process the supplements you devour.

At the point when wellness fans and competitors talk about intermittent fasting, they are typically discussing an eating program that is different from the intermittent fasting depicted in the logical writing. Under research center conditions, guineas pigs devoured no calories during the fasting time frame. In reality, this can cause issues since we need to work grinding away and at home. Individuals who eat on an intermittent fasting plan, for the most part, refrain from eating during the fasting time frame yet get a few calories as low-calorie refreshments, for example, espresso or tea.

This isn't the main way that this present reality variant of intermittent fasting veers off from the research facility rendition.

Do a snappy Internet scan for intermittent fasting timetable, and you'll see about the same number of varieties as there are individuals who adhere to an intermittent fasting plan. Huge numbers of these individuals have extraordinary examples of overcoming adversity, which delineates how helpful this sort of calendar can be. Intermittent fasting is effortlessly adjusted to meet your requirements.

It may sound somewhat outrageous to propose fasting for sixteen hours every day and eating for just eight hours, however in all actuality, and you are now fasting for six to eight hours consistently on the off chance that you are getting the prescribed measure of rest. That is up to half of your fasting time on the off chance that you utilize a 16/8 calendar, which most likely makes the possibility of confronting a sixteen-hour fast considerably less overwhelming.

Eating on an intermittent fasting plan doesn't imply that you are cutting calories or supplements, but instead that you get the entirety of your supplements during your eating period. Being in a fasting state will neither reason you to lose bulk, nor will it weaken your capacity to fabricate new muscle. You can even train in a fasting state.

Reexamining Common Sense

Intermittent fasting depends on the possibility that the aggregate sum of supplements that you devour is a higher priority than guaranteeing they are conveyed on the correct occasions.

We are told over, and over that creation, sure your body has a consistent inventory of protein and amino acids is the ideal approach to guarantee that it can assemble muscles most effectively. In any case, there is proof this can really shield your body from building muscle as proficiently as possible.

The possibility that a consistent wellspring of protein is expected to keep your body in an anabolic state is defective. Eating high-protein meals a few hours separated is probably not going to animate extra muscle development on the grounds that the corrosive amino levels in your body don't drain as fast as your protein levels do. Essentially, your body becomes desensitized to elevated levels of protein over the long haul. Meals dispersed further separated can recondition your body's affectability to protein and amino acids.

The abatement in muscle protein blend is only one manner by which the six meals for each day program is flawed. Another imperfection is the impact that visits meals have on your body's capacity to consume fat, which is a significant procedure for individuals whose objective is to get slender and for bodybuilders. Furnishing your body with a consistent inventory of vitality implies that it won't have to consume fat, which it possibly does when it has drained the entirety of your different wellsprings of vitality.

The six meals for each day program are situated partially on the possibility that you will feel less ravenous between meals, making you more averse to gorge each time you do eat and less inclined to nibble on unhealthy foods between meals. Be that as it may, this can likewise be broken much of the time.

Individuals who got one high-protein meal instead of five littler meals felt less craving later on and ate less at their next meal. This recommends visit meals may make you bound to eat additional calories, which is something contrary to the expected impact of diminishing your craving.

Notwithstanding, conceivably negatively affecting your body, and the outcomes you get from working out, eating six meals daily can get monotonous. Halting what you are doing each a few hours to set up a meal doesn't typically fit into the vast majority's calendars. Numerous individuals on a preparation diet dedicate one whole day every week – for the most part toward the end of the week – to set up the entirety of their meals for the up and coming week. Not exclusively would this be able to take up a whole Sunday, yet the expense of purchasing and supplanting plastic compartments to convey your meals can likewise be restrictive for this sort of meal planning.

The most effective method to Schedule Your Fasts

There are no hard standards with respect to how you plan your fasting periods and sustained periods. There are basic rules that individuals by and large follow when beginning an intermittent fasting program, yet perhaps the best favorable position of this sort of program is that it is adjustable. You can change your eating timetable to accommodate your way of life as opposed to organizing your whole day around your meals. This signifies, if one fasting/encouraging timetable doesn't accommodate your daily practice, do a little research for recommendations on what transforms you can make.

The vast majority on an intermittent fasting plan utilizes a 16/8 timetable, which means sixteen hours fasting and eight hours bolstering. This is commonly the most straightforward calendar, to begin with since around half of your fasting time is during rest, which is the point at which you would fast at any rate. The sustaining time frame will, in general, be among early afternoon and 8 P.M.

You should pick whether you would want to work out while fasting or subsequent to having eaten. On the off chance that you cling to the early afternoon to 8 P.M. eating plan, this essentially comes down to whether you turn out in the first part of the day or evening. Recall that you can change your timetable to oblige your necessities. In the event that you want to turn out toward the beginning of the day subsequent to eating, you can change your fasting and bolstering periods to permit you to do this.

Preparing during Fasting

Fasted preparing requires a few enhancements to keep your body in an anabolic state. The body utilizes amino acids for vitality in the event that you are preparing without a pre-exercise meal. Your enhancements for fasted preparation ought to incorporate glutamine and an extended chain amino corrosive enhancement.

Dealing with the early afternoon to 8 P.M. sustaining plan, you fast from 8 P.M. until 10 or 11 A.M. Now, take your glutamine and BCAA enhancements, and afterward do your exercise. Contingent upon to what extent your exercise keeps going, this will put your post-exercise meal at around early afternoon or 1 P.M. What number of meals you decide to gobble during your encouraging period is up to you, however, recall that eating less as often as possible can hold your yearning within proper limits and can support your body's capacity to integrate muscle.

Preparing during Feeding

On the off chance that you like to turn out subsequent to eating, you can plan your exercise to fall in the early evening (early afternoon to 1 P.M.) or toward the evening (around 4 P.M.) If your exercise is for the most part in the early evening, eat your pre-exercise meal around early afternoon, do your exercise, and afterward eat your different meals.

For a mid-evening exercise, eat your first meal around early afternoon and your pre-exercise meal at 3 P.M. On the off chance that you want to eat a post-exercise meal inside an hour of working out, you can do as such.

Adjusting Your Calorie Intake

The main genuine principles about intermittent fasting include a few parts of when and how you get your calories and macronutrients.

On the off chance that you train while fasting, the calorie check of your BCAA supplement ought to be tallied toward your complete calorie mean the day, in spite of the fact that it doesn't end your fasting period. Individuals on intermittent fasting plan normally distribute fifty calories for their fasting period to take into account things like enhancements or refreshments. This implies you can, in any case, take cream and sugar in your espresso or tea, regardless of whether it is during your fasting period.

On the off chance that you eat a pre-exercise meal, it is ideal for keeping it light. Your meal ought to incorporate a protein source like poultry or fish, some foods grown from the ground, all signifying 400-600 calories. This will give you the protein and complex starches that are oftentimes suggested for pre-exercise meals. On the off chance that you do eat a pre-exercise meal, the BCAA supplements prescribed for fasting exercises are most likely redundant. You might need to take them in any case, since having an overflow of BCAAs may even now be helpful.

Your post-exercise meal is the best time to expend a large portion of your sugars and calories. About portion of your absolute calories for the day ought to be eaten during your post-exercise meal.

Changing in accordance with Intermittent Fasting

One of the most troublesome deterrents to overcome when you initially start intermittent fasting is the manner in which you have adapted your body to anticipate visit meals. Your body's creation of ghrelin, the hormone that makes you feel hunger, adjusts to your general encouraging calendar. This implies you need to permit it to acclimate to fewer meals, which can take some time.

Following your calorie and macronutrient intake can help facilitate the change from your six meal timetable to an intermittent fasting plan. On the off chance that you have been on a preparation diet for any period of time, you are presumably no outsider to recording what you eat, or in any event, monitoring it with a PC program or cell phone application. This will assist you with changing over your six little meals into a couple of bigger ones to accommodate your intermittent fasting way of life.

Intermittent fasting is very much adjusted to any calendar, which is most likely why it has such wide intrigue. Huge numbers of the individuals who change to an intermittent fasting plan rush to discuss what an alleviation it isn't to need to invest such a lot of energy getting ready and eating food. Since you never again need to worry about food, make sure to be adaptable once in a while.

You may have a family occasion that includes eating sooner or later during your fasting period. Some portion of the intrigue of intermittent fasting is that you never again need to structure your life to suit your dietary patterns, so don't worry about eating when you ought to fast on these events.

WHAT IS INTERMITTENT FASTING FOR WOMEN OVER 60

The term intermittent fasting (IF) can apply to any number of totally different dietary conventions. In contrast to "genuine" fasting, where no calories are devoured for a supported timeframe, intermittent fasting frequently permits a few calories even on "fast" days, and those days are scattered with typical calorie "feed" days.

Substitute day fasting (ADF) includes expending from 0 to 25 percent of every day calorie needs on interchange days, with ordinary encouraging in the middle. The 5:2 IF diet is comparative, then again, actually 25 percent of calories are devoured on only two non-continuous "fast" days of the week, with typical benefiting from the other five days.

At last, there is time-limited sustaining (TRF), which truly isn't fasting in any way, however where ordinary encouraging is confined to a generally brief timeframe (between 10 a.m. what's more, 6 p.m., for instance), on a continuous premise.

Intermittent fasting (IF) portrays an example of eating that cycles between times of fasting and typical eating.

The most widely recognized methods remember fasting for substitute days, day by day 16-hour fasts, or fasting for 24 hours, two days per week. With the end goal of this digital book, the term intermittent fasting will be utilized to portray all regimens.

In contrast to most diets, intermittent fasting doesn't include the following calories or macronutrients. Indeed, there are no necessities about what foods to eat or avoid, making it all the more a way of life than a diet.

Numerous individuals utilize intermittent fasting to shed pounds as it is a basic, advantageous, and successful approach to eat less and diminish body fat.

It might likewise help decrease the danger of heart illness and diabetes, protect bulk, and improve mental prosperity.

Additionally, this dietary example can assist spare with timing in the kitchen as you have fewer meals to plan, plan, and cook.

INTERMITTENT FASTING CAN ALSO BE DEFINED AS....

Intermittent fasting is an eating plan where you cycle between times of eating and fasting.

It doesn't utter a word about which foods to eat, yet rather when you ought to eat them.

There are diverse types of intermittent fasting methods, all of which split the day or week into eating periods and fasting periods.

A great many people effectively "fast" consistently, while they rest. Intermittent fasting can be as basic as expanding that fast somewhat more.

You can do this by skipping breakfast, eating your first meal around early afternoon, and your last meal at 8 pm.

At that point, you're actually fasting for 16 hours consistently and limiting your eating to an 8-hour eating window. This most common type of intermittent fasting, known as the 16/8 technique.

In spite of what you may think, intermittent fasting is entirely simple to do. Numerous individuals report feeling good and having more vitality during a fast.

Yearning is generally not unreasonably enormous of an issue, in spite of the fact that it very well may be an issue at the outset, while your body is becoming accustomed to not eating for expanded timeframes.

No food is permitted during the fasting time frame, yet you can drink water, espresso, tea, and other non-caloric refreshments.
A few types of intermittent fasting permit modest quantities of low-calorie foods during the fasting time frame.

Taking enhancements is, for the most part, permitted while fasting, as long as there are no calories in them.

Intermittent fasting (or "IF") is an eating plan where you cycle between times of eating and fasting. It is an extremely well-known health and wellness pattern, with research to back it up.

BENEFITS OF INTERMITTENT FASTING FOR WOMEN OVER 60

The general benefits that propel women over 60years towards taking up intermittent fasting include:

- Enhanced slender muscle development

- Increase in vitality

- Continuous weight loss

- An increased cell stress response

- Reduced aggravation and oxidative pressure

- Improvement in insulin affectability in women who are overweight

- Enhanced intellectual capacity because of expanded nerve development factor creation

The most significant and prompt advantage you put on with the IF is weight loss. Different benefits incorporate fix of the cells, improved emotional wellness, and diminished insulin obstruction.

Presently returning to the weight-loss impact. It happens in an accompanying manner:

- The intake of standard meals under a shorter time span leaves you feeling satisfied for the entire day.

- The full inclination keeps you from eating in the middle of meals.

- During the course of fasting, the body goes into the fasted state. This state cultivates fat-consuming, which had been distant in the fed state.

- The body goes into the fasted stage in around 8-12 hours after the last meal you take.

- This is the motivation behind why you can lose fat without changing the sort and amount of food you eat and the recurrence of your exercises.

1. Weight Loss

The most well-known search out the advantage of intermittent fasting is weight loss. The odds are acceptable; this is the fundamental explanation you're understanding this. Yet, continue perusing in light of the fact that there are a lot more that you may not be acquainted with.

As we get more established, our digestion systems delayed down, toss in peri-menopause or menopause and progressively fat beginnings gathering in territories where we don't need it, and intermittent fasting can help.

Corpulent grown-ups who followed a substitute day intermittent fasting plan lost as much as 13 pounds over about two months. Be cautious on the off chance that you attempt this strategy, since it additionally has its negative focuses, for example, eating a lot when that you're not fasting.

Not exclusively does intermittent fasting advance fat loss, you likewise hold muscle while fasting not at all like typical calorie prohibitive diets.

Intermittent fasting may support weight loss through a few systems.

To start with, limiting your meals and snacks to an exacting time window may normally diminish your calorie intake, which can help weight loss.

Intermittent fasting may likewise expand levels of norepinephrine, a hormone, and synapse that can support your digestion to build calorie consuming for the duration of the day.

Moreover, this eating example may lessen levels of insulin, a hormone associated with glucose the executives. Diminished levels can knock up fat consumption to advance weight loss.

Some examination even shows that intermittent fasting can enable your body to hold bulk more adequately than calorie limitation, which may expand its allure.

As indicated by one audit, intermittent fasting may diminish body weight by up to 8% and decline body fat by up to 16% over 3–12 weeks.

Cooperative energy with keto

At the point when combined with the ketogenic diet, intermittent fasting can accelerate ketosis and enhance weight loss.

The keto diet, which is high in fats yet low in carbs, is intended to launch ketosis.

Ketosis is a metabolic express that powers your body to consume fat for fuel rather than carbs. This happens when your body is denied of glucose, which is its primary wellspring of vitality.

Joining intermittent fasting with the keto diet can enable your body to enter ketosis faster to amplify results. It can, in like manner, alleviate a portion of the reactions that frequently happen when beginning this diet, including the keto influenza, which is described by queasiness, cerebral pains, and weakness.

Intermittent fasting can build weight loss by boosting fat consumption and digestion. At the point when utilized pair with the ketogenic diet, it might assist speed with increasing ketosis to amplify weight loss.

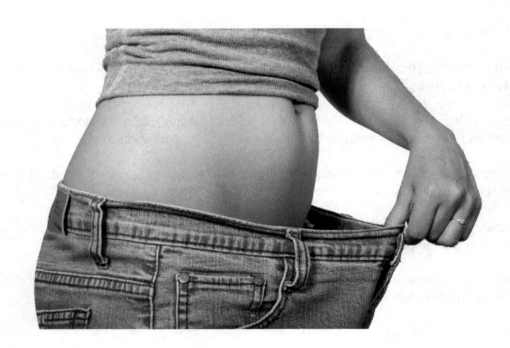

Cleans Defective Cells

Intermittent fasting advances autophagy, which is where the body disposes of cells that have a more serious danger of getting contaminated or destructive. Faulty cells that are not working at top execution can prompt fastened maturing, Alzheimer's malady, and type 2 diabetes.

The fixing procedure happens going full speed ahead as the body doesn't need to concentrate on the assimilation of food. It can focus on cell fix completely. This procedure is called autophagy.

Consequently, fasting assists with relieving or right now your body and causes it to work appropriately.

This resembles spring cleaning for your body, disposing of the "broken" cells. It makes room for healthy cells and expands your health and dynamic quality.

Fasting makes our cells become stronger to harm without weight loss. What's more, do these benefits rely upon the impermanent pressure that fasting causes in our cells?

Intermittent Fasting May Have Anti-Aging Benefits

Researchers have been taking a gander at the conceivable health benefits of calorie limitation for a considerable length of time.

A conspicuous hypothesis recommends these health benefits are identified with the drop in glucose that outcomes from fasting, which pushes our cells to work more diligently to use different types of vitality.

Rhesus monkeys eating just 70% of their ordinary caloric intake have been appeared to live any longer and are a lot healthier at more established ages. This enemy of maturing benefits has additionally been found in creatures that are put on an intermittent fasting diet, shifting back and forth between long periods of typical eating and days where calories are limited.

What isn't clear, however, is the reason intermittent fasting appears to have an advantage in the battle against maturing. This inquiry is muddled by the way that in all examinations acted in individuals, and fasting prompted weight loss. The health benefits of weight loss may be overshadowing different benefits acquired from fasting alone.

One way that our cells can become harmed is the point at which they experience oxidative pressure. Also, forestalling or fixing cell harm from oxidative pressure is useful against maturing. This pressure happens when there is a higher-than-typical creation of free radicals, for example, responsive oxygen species. These are insecure particles that convey exceptionally receptive electrons.

At the point when one of these free radicals experiences another particle, it might either surrender an electron or take another electron. This can bring about a fast chain response from particle to atom, shaping all the more free radicals, which can break separated associations between iotas inside significant segments of the phone, similar to the phone film, fundamental proteins, or even DNA. Enemies of oxidants work by moving the required electrons to balance out the free radicals before they can do any damage.

In spite of the fact that fasting appears to enable our cells to battle harm from this procedure, it isn't clear precisely how that occurs.

Free radicals can be created by inadequately working mitochondria (the powerhouses of the cell). The switch between eating typically and fasting makes cells briefly experience lower-than-regular degrees of (glucose), and they are compelled to start utilizing different wellsprings of less promptly accessible vitality, similar to unsaturated fats. This can make the cells turn on endurance procedures to evacuate the unhealthy mitochondria and supplant them with healthy ones over time, subsequently lessening the creation of free radicals in the long haul.

It may likewise be valid that fasting itself brings about a little increment in free extreme creation right off the bat during fasting.

The cells may react by expanding their degrees of common enemies of oxidants to battle against future free radicals. Also, albeit free radicals are usually observed as unsafe due to their capacity to harm our phones, they may be significant momentary signs for our body right now, cells to adapt better to increasingly extreme burdens that may come later on.

Intermittent fasting can keep your body more youthful, broaden your life expectancy, and improve your overall health, another Harvard University study proposes. ... Some examination has indicated that intermittent fasting offers no benefits over everyday dietary limitations. However, the creature considers have discovered that it was connected to longer life expectancies.

3. Forestalls Breast Cancer Recurrence

A more extended time of fasting is a decent technique to decrease bosom malignant growth repeat. This investigation of bosom malignancy survivors who didn't eat for in any event 12 and half hours overnight had a 36 percent decrease in the danger of their bosom disease returning.

Intermittent fasting can assist your body with resisting the advancement of the disease. At the point when we fast, blood glucose levels decline, and the body begins to utilize our fat stores. This secures against the improvement of malignancy in a few different ways:

- Being overweight expands the danger of creating a wide range of sorts of disease, one so by basically getting in shape through intermittent fasting, we can decrease our malignant growth risk.

- **Fasting triggers a change from development to fix.** At the point when our body changes to fix mode (named autophagy), any harmed cells or parts of cells are stalled, and their bits reused to make new, well-working cells. This especially influences cells, which may turn harmful.

- Fasting can likewise diminish the measure of the hormone, insulin-like development factor 1 (IGF-1), which has been seen as related to an expanded malignancy hazard. A few people appear to have especially high IGF-1 levels, and there is, by all accounts, an unbalanced number of malignancy patients with high IGF-1 levels.

- The decline in blood glucose keeps malignant growth cells from fuel. Malignant cells, for the most part, can't utilize fats or ketones for fuel – they utilize just glucose – thus, though our typical cells can oversee fine and dandy with fats or ketones, the diseased cells are famished and can't develop.

4.Brings down Your Risk of Developing Type 2 Diabetes

- Two diabetes regularly creates in individuals over the age of 45. The Centers for Disease Control and Prevention express that in excess of 30 million Americans have diabetes (around 1 out of 10), and 90%-95% of them have type 2 diabetes.

- Are entirely startling insights.

- Can create Type 2 diabetes when your cells don't regularly react to insulin. Insulin is a hormone secreted in the gut by the pancreas, which permits cells to assimilate and utilize glucose (sugar) as vitality.

- In the event that you become insulin safe, your cells aren't open to insulin and can't ingest glucose. Sugar at that point develops in your circulatory system, which can be dangerous. All together for your body to get the glucose out of the circulation system, it stores it as fat.

- Fasting to be related to decreases in glucose, insulin, and upgrades to insulin affectability.

- Fasting could offer insurance against type 2 diabetes by decreasing the gathering of fat around the pancreas, German specialists have said.

- Fasting includes fasting for specific periods, which can fluctuate long. One of the most notable types of organized fasting is the 5:2 diet, which includes utilizing fasting to accomplish an exceptionally low-calorie intake on two days of the week. Elective renditions of fasting incorporate constraining food intake to inside an eight-hour window every day.

- Has recently been appeared to bring down HbA1c in individuals with type 2 diabetes, just as empowering weight loss. Overweight mice built to be in danger of type 2 diabetes took a gander at the effect that confining meals at specific times had on fat in the pancreas.

- Aggregations outside the fat tissue, for example, in the liver, muscles, or even bones, negatively affect these organs and the whole body. What effect fat cells have inside the pancreas has not been clear as of recently,"

5. Lifts Brain Health

- Fasting can smother irritation in the cerebrum. Irritation is related to neurological conditions, for example, Alzheimer's sickness, Parkinson's infection, and stroke.

- One of these procedures (protein saving, a decrease of irritation, autophagy, and increment of BDNF creation) advantage our cerebrum. From one viewpoint, they decrease the harm to synapses by, for instance, holding down incendiary responses and disposing of waste in mind. Then again, they additionally animate appropriate mind work, by advancing cell fix and adding to the arrangement of new synapses and associations between them, in this way encouraging correspondence inside the cerebrum. BDNF specifically adds to this structured procedure, and shortages right now been connected to psychological issues during maturing, for example, dementia. So IF has a neuroprotective impact and along these lines adds to healthy maturing.

6. Improves Heart Health

- Fasting can prompt a decrease in pulse, heart rate, cholesterol, and triglycerides in people and creatures.

- Hard to determine what impact fasting has on your heart health on the grounds that numerous individuals who routinely fast frequently do as such for health or strict reasons. These individuals, for the most part, tend to not smoke, which additionally can diminish heart ailment chance.

- In any case, in any event, one investigation has shown that individuals who follow a fasting diet may have preferred heart health over individuals who don't. This might be on the grounds that individuals who routinely fast show restraint over what number of calories they eat and drink, and this conduct may convert into weight control and better eating decisions when they aren't fasting.

- Fasting and better heart health may likewise be connected to the manner in which your body processes cholesterol and sugar. Ordinary fasting can diminish your low-thickness lipoprotein, or "terrible," cholesterol. It's additionally felt that fasting may improve the manner in which your body processes sugar. This can decrease your danger of putting on weight and treating diabetes, which are both hazard factors for a heart ailment.

7.Permits Your Body to Heal

- The point when you're continually eating, you're not giving your body and your cells the time they have to rest. They need this opportunity to fix themselves, or to dispose of those cells that the body feels may get tainted or destructive.

- Consider your pour stomach related framework continually working. Give it a rest!

- cells

- Fix procedure happens going full speed ahead as the body doesn't need to concentrate on the absorption of food. It can focus on cell fix completely. This procedure is called autophagy.

- This way, fasting assists with restoring or right now your body and causes it to work appropriately.

- consistent discernment

- The significant advantage of IF is that you can concentrate on assignments better and finish a significant segment of your outstanding task at hand in the while in the fasting state.

- insulin obstruction

- Obstruction happens when you continually have high glucose. This prompts the powerlessness of your body to follow up on the sugar content in the blood and separate it.

- The point when you take up intermittent fasting, it encourages you to monitor the glucose level.

- Condition is additionally activated because of elements like raised circulatory strain, inertia, hereditary qualities, ill-advised diet, stoutness, or overabundance body weight.

- In any case, other than all the benefits, there are sure contemplations to think about.

- First is the fasting stage that causes the creation of leptin and ghrelin – the appetite hormones. Be that as it may, as women over 60 give intermittent fasting some time, they report feeling less ravenous over the long haul.

- The second factor in intermittent fasting for women is the fasting debilitates the conceptive limit, so it isn't prescribed for pregnant women to fastly. On the off chance that a lady who fasts neglects to devour enough calories, she may have some fruitfulness issues. In any case, IF is done accurately, there's no compelling reason to stress. In the wake of losing some overweight women may even improve their richness.

DISADVANTAGES OF INTERMITTENT FASTING FOR WOMEN OVER 60

- Decide to fast for an assortment of reasons, regardless of whether they are identified with health, weight loss, accounts, or religion. Fasting can go from juice-just fasts to fasts that bar all food and liquid, for example, dry fasting. While fasts could once in a while have some health benefits, they could likewise be risky. Fasting has contrary effects in the short and long haul and has adverse impacts for some individuals, including the individuals who need to shed pounds. At last, the impacts of swearing off food fluctuate to a great extent, dependent on the person who is fasting.

Management

- It can really be hindering for weight the board, as indicated by enrolled dietitians on MayoClinic.com. After a time of fasting, People will come in general ache for starchier foods, with more fatty substances. Sugars are the body's favored wellspring of fuel. Extraordinary appetite likewise makes you pack on a greater number of calories than are healthy for the body to expand at a time. At last, fasting can switch the planned impacts of weight the board plan.

- Side Effects

- Are some transient symptoms of fasting—these incorporate migraines, tipsiness, discombobulation, exhaustion, low circulatory strain, and irregular heart rhythms. Individuals who are fasting may encounter a weakened capacity to lead certain errands, for example, work hardware or drive a vehicle. Fasting could likewise cause flare-ups of specific conditions, for example, gout or gallstones. Fasting could debilitate the body's capacity to retain certain meds or even adjust tranquilize connections in the body.

Haul Side Effects

- Has hindering effects in the long haul also. Not exclusively can fasting harm the insusceptible framework, it can likewise contrarily influence a significant number of the body's organs, including the liver and kidneys. Fasting could meddle with substantial crucial capacity. Keeping away from eating could likewise be conceivably hazardous in people who are now malnourished, for instance, malignant growth patients. It's even feasible for fasting to bring about death when the body's put away vitality is completely exhausted.

Fasting

- There are numerous methods of fasting, dry fasting - or avoiding all liquid and food intake - is especially risky. Dry fasting can rapidly prompt parchedness and passing in simply an issue of days. The American Cancer Society reports the health effect of dry fasting shifts to a great extent, dependent on the individual and setting. Factors, for example, heat, substantial effort, and traded off health, can make dry fasting deadly in simply a question of hours.

- Past, Intermittent Fasting has a clouded side as well. One of the most evident disadvantages is getting profoundly fixated on following the intermittent fasting plan correctly. An individual would get inflexible in eating, especially now and again, he/she has fixed prior. For instance, in the event that you have intended to take the primary meal of the day at 12:00 pm, and you are starving by 11:60 am, you may delay eating for 10 minutes. Such over the top dietary patterns are adverse to one's mental prosperity.

Lethargy...

- A significant factor related to the hurtful impacts of intermittent fasting is the hunger not being successfully fulfilled. Albeit an individual is genuinely full, he/she will be enticed to eat more. This conduct prompts over-eating, and it nearly murders the hidden motivation behind getting in shape by beginning intermittent fasting in any case.

- Section of this terrible clouded side of intermittent fasting is the (purportedly) definitely diminished vitality levels during the previous pieces of the day. This outcome in an individual inclination apathetic and torpid during work and furthermore causes decreased fixation levels that can influence one's capacity to do everyday exercises.

Hunger

- A normal symptom of fasting diets is that they can modify the parity of your hormones. In particular, the decrease in leptin (which causes you to feel full), and the expansion in cortisol (which can bring about your body being under more pressure, and accordingly a stop in weight loss). A Study on fasting indicated female understudies leptin diminished by as much as 75%, and their cortisol expanded by as quite a bit of 60% after the fasting time of the investigation. Expanded cortisol can likewise bring about changes in the menstrual cycle for women.

Imbalances

- Fatty people (who have less weight to lose), and those with effectively dynamic ways of life are the ones well on the way to encounter this con to intermittent fasting. As referenced in the past point, the interruption in hormones can prompt sporadic menstrual cycles for women, diminished testosterone in men, and furthermore to more instances of a sleeping disorder and higher announced feelings of anxiety in all investigation members of any sex. Corpulent people who participate in intermittent fasting are bound to encounter benefits and have a higher level of fat loss over the fasting time frame.

- Very well may be derived from the models over that we can't announce climate Intermittent Fasting is 'acceptable' or 'terrible,' it is altogether up to your circumstance, current health, and body fat rate. In case you intend to take on an intermittent fasting schedule, it ought to be controlled so that its negative outcomes are as negligible as could be allowed. There are different types of intermittent fasting accessible, for instance, fasting just on ends of the week, fasting elective days, it doesn't need to be something you do each day of the week!

TYPES OF INTERMITTENT FASTING FOR WOMEN OVER 60

The most part, they are heaps of intermittent fasting for women to rehearse, in the interim, there are a concise, i.e., six significant types of intermittent fasting for women above 5o years old.

We proceed with the six significant types of intermittent fasting for women above 5o years; we will, as a matter of first importance, research and experience the by and large types of intermittent fasting that women practice.

Are various reasons and methods for doing intermittent fasting, yet it's basic to isolate a bit of the guideline stating.

Fasting – the exhibit of denying food confirmation or anything that has calories for a particular time allotment. Normally, some non-caloric beverages and water are allowed.

Intermittent Fasting – doing fasting intermittently and joining shorter fasts into your step by step plan.

Extended Fasting – the exhibition of fasting for a drawn-out time span for additional clinical advantages. It will, in general, be cultivated for a significant long time or even weeks.

Time-Restricted Feeding – the exhibition of constraining your regular food usage inside a particular time window. This will improve the circadian state of mind and general prosperity.

Around, people doing intermittent fasting are basically time-constraining their food and less fasting. To group something like a fast, it would need to prop up for over 24 hours since that is the spot most by far of the benefits start to kick in.

direct – you just quit eating – yet for perfect results, you'd have to concentrate on these different types of intermittent fasting recorded underneath

24-Hour Fasting

It is the fundamental technique for doing intermittent fasting – you fast for around 24 hours, and a short time later has a meal. It doesn't have to suggest that you truly experience a day without eating. Simply eat around evening time, fast all through the next day, and eat again.

Can even have your food at the 23-hour check and eat it inside an hour. The idea is to compel a more prominent caloric deficiency for the day and undereat. Most of the benefits will be vain if you, regardless of everything, crevasse and put on weight.

Degree and once in a while, you can fastly depend upon your physical condition and imperativeness necessities.

A fit person who prepares and exercises constantly would require to some degree progressively visit eating and less fasting.

An overweight person who is latent and endeavors to lose some weight could fast as long as they can until they lose the overabundance weight.

And skipping suppers have gotten degenerate in the propelled food condition since you can eat anything wherever. It's in like manner the 'F-articulation' of the health business. In any case, fasting should be viewed as the easiest and fastest strategy for getting fit as a fiddle.

16/8 Intermittent Fasting

- Practiced the 16/8 style intermittent fasting a great deal.

- 16:8 intermittent fasting was advanced by Martin Berkhan of Leangains. It's cultivated for improving fat loss while up 'til now having the choice to get ready hard.

- Fundamental – you fast for 16 hours and eat your food inside 8. What number of dinners you have inside that time length is irrelevant, yet whatever else than 2-3 isn't significant.

- In my own view, this should be the base fasting length to concentrate on by everybody reliably. There is no physical inspiration to eat any sooner than that, and the restriction has various benefits.

- A large number of individuals believe that it is more straightforward to post-pone breakfast by two or three hours and eat around early evening. You don't should be insane, and that is demanding about breaking the fast The idea is simply to reduce the proportion of time we spend in a continued state and excessively fastly a large portion of the day.

The Warrior Diet

- Warrior Diet is proposed by Ori Hofmekler. He jabbers about the benefits of fasting on pressure change through the miracle of hormesis.

- Not simply improves your body's physical condition and ability to bear upsetting conditions yet, moreover, hones your mental attitude and outlook.

- Warrior Diet talks about old warriors like Spartans and Romans who may remain genuinely unique all through the entire day and generally eat around evening time. During light, they would stroll around with 40 pounds of rigging, produce fortresses, and bear the warming sun of the Mediterranean simultaneously getting just a few eats of food as it were. Around evening time, they would have a huge supper contained stews, meat, bits of bread, and different things.

- The Warrior Diet, you fast for around 20 hours, have a short high power exercise, and eat your food inside 4 hours. All things considered, it would fuse either two more diminutive meals with a break-in or one single colossal eating experience.

One Meal a Day OMAD

- Meal a Day Diet is otherwise called OMAD. You basically eat once consistently, and it's done.

- OMAD, you regularly fast around 21-23 hours and eat your food inside a 1-2 hour time allotment. This is remarkable for dieting since you can feel full and satisfied while up 'til now staying at a caloric setback.

- It is unprecedented for losing fat; be that as it may, not ideal for muscle improvement because of the compelled time for protein blend and anabolism. It's a very moderate method.

- inclusion in intermittent fasting following 7 years of fasting

36-Hour Fasting

- People would much of the time go a couple of days without eating, yet they suffer and even thrived. Nowadays, the typical individual can't skip breakfast, likewise head to rest hungry.

- For over 24 hours is the spot, all the charm begins. The more you stay in a fasted state and experience imperativeness hardship, the more your body is constrained to trigger its life expectancy pathways that help to actuate fat stores, bolster juvenile microorganisms, and reuse old wrecked cell material through the system of autophagy.

- It takes, at any rate, a day to see gigantic signs of autophagy, yet you can speed it up by eating low carb before starting the fast, rehearsing on an unfilled stomach, and exhausting some homegrown teas that enliven this strategy.

- For 36 hours isn't that irksome truly. You fundamentally eat the previous night, don't eat anything in the initial segment of the day, lunch nor evening, head to rest in a fasted state, wake up the next day, fast a few hours more, and start eating again.

- That makes the fasting more straightforward are gleaming water, mineral water, dull coffee, green tea, and some homegrown teas.

1. 48-Hour Fasting

- The case you recently made it to the 36-hour mark, by then, why not just fast for the entire 48 hours.

- It is only irksome during the vital change to organize. After you cross the crevasse, which generally occurs around your normal dinner time, by then, it gets straightforward.

- The point when your body goes into increasingly significant ketosis and institutes autophagy, you will cover hunger, feel mentally totally clear, and have greater essentialness and center intrigue.

- The most problematic bit of any comprehensive fast is around the 24-hour mark. If it is possible for you to fall asleep and wake up the next day, by then, you've set yourself prepared for fasting for a significant period of time and days with no issues. You essentially need to get over this hidden obstruction.

- The sack hungry sounds disturbing; in any case, that is what a huge bit of the absolute masses is doing each day. It causes you to contemplate your own fortune and be logically thankful for your food.

Expanded Fasting for 3-7 Days

- For 48-hours would give you a short lift in autophagy and some fat consuming; be that as it may, to genuinely get the medicinal benefits of fasting, you'd have to fast for 3+ days.

- It has been shown that 72-hours of fasting can reset the protected structure in mice]. This turns on pathways of undifferentiated hematopoietic creatures, which makes platelets and advances opposition.

- For 3-5 days is moreover the perfect timeframe for autophagy likewise, after which you begin to see unavoidable losses. Fasting for 7 days and past isn't required overall. Most people don't need to fast any more drawn out than that since you may start losing fit muscle tissue.

- Fitting for people to concentrate on 3-4 of these widely inclusive fasts every year to propel cell recovering and clear out the body. Notwithstanding eating a strong eating routine and not having any lousy sustenance, I, regardless of everything, do it considering the dazzling benefits.

- The case you're overweight, or you experience the evil impacts of some illness, by then longer fasts can really help you with mending yourself. Fast for 3-5 days, have a little refeed, and repeat the methodology until significant.

Alternate Day Fasting

- Are also advances toward like The 5:2 Diet and Alternate Day Fasting, which join fasting, be that as it may, license the use of around 600 calories on significant stretches of abstention. Those restricted amounts of calories are only for extending consistency.

- To eat at an extraordinary caloric constraint won't grant the total of the physiological benefits of fasting to kick in totally. You would expand a segment of the impacts; in any case, an absolute limitation is fundamental all the more convincing for both your physiology and mind science.

- The FMD which also means the Fasting Mimicking Diet have their place, and they can be used every so often. Commonly, they're supported to people who can't fast like the old or some restorative patients.

- Everybody can get fast. It's basically that some can't intellectually manage the weight and to not eat. That is the spot these fasting impersonating diets and exchange day fasting shows can help.

Fasting Mimicking Diet (FMD)

- Fasting imitating diet has been seemed to reduce circulatory strain, lower insulin, and cover IGF-1, all of which have positive benefits on life length. Regardless, these impacts are likely an immediate consequence of the outrageous caloric restriction.

- The Fasting Mimicking Diet, you'd eat low protein, moderate carb, moderate fat foods like mushroom soup, olives, kale wafers, and some nut bars. The idea is to, regardless, give you something to eat while keeping the calories as low as would be reasonable. In any case, again, this is basically to satisfy the people's mental needs to eat.

- With zero calories would be logically effective, and it will truly keep up more muscle tissue by staying in increasingly significant ketosis.

- Thwart unwanted loss of lean mass; you can change the macronutrient extents of the FMD and make them more ketogenic by cutting down the carbs and extending the fat possibly.

Protein Sparing Modified Fasting

- Protein-saving altered fast (PSMF) is a low carb, low fat, high protein sort of diet that helps with getting increasingly fit genuinely fast while propelling muscle upkeep.

- Thin mass is a significant matter of stress for people who are into health, especially in case they're endeavoring to do intermittent fasting.

- It is a catabolic stressor that will, over the long haul, lead to muscle loss; notwithstanding, the rate is a great deal of lower than people may speculate. To shield that from happening, you have to stay in ketosis and lower the body's enthusiasm for glucose. Right when ketones are accessible, the essential for isolating muscle into essentialness reduces on a very basic level.

- PSMF is absolutely going to keep up more muscle than the fasting reflecting diet, yet there's the danger of being dismissed out of ketosis on the from chance that you eat an abundance of protein right now orchestrating yourself to muscle catabolism.

- Avoid muscle loss on the protein-saving changed fastly; you have to keep protein moderate around 0.8-1.0 g/lb of body weight and addition your fat a smidgen. By and large, you'd even now stay under 1000 calories every day.

Fat Fasting

- The fasting Physiology and the ketogenic diet are in a general sense equivalent to, and both of them start the metabolic state of ketosis.

- When you're dieting i.e in ketosis, you're using fat and ketones as a basic fuel source as opposed to glucose. This enables you to pick up induction to essentialness throughout each and every day in light of the fact that you'll be consuming your own body fat.

- Simply fat during a fast ala fat fasting won't show you out of ketosis. It likely raises your ketones hardly. Nevertheless, it will smother autophagy a bit.

- A couple of types of autophagy like chaperone-interceded autophagy can safeguard ketones and keep up their belongings; be that as it may, it's not as amazing as macroautophagy, which requires the restraint from all calories.

- Fat fast can be used for propelling adherence and guaranteeing you don't stop mostly through.

- Fat fasting, you can have a pinch of Bulletproof coffee, 1-2 tsp of MCT oil, or some margarine anyway anything with carbs or protein in it like bone stock, coconut milk, overwhelming cream, coconut water, or the like will break the fast.
- Bone Broth Fasting

- Soup fasting is so far a sensible option for widened fasting in case it causes you nonsensically fast for additional.

- The stock has some amino acids in it that really can quell autophagy yet in case you just refreshment a lone cup; by then, you'll find in all probability smother autophagy for just two or three hours and get again into it fastly.

- You're doing fasting for autophagy; by then, you have to use bone soup and different calories when in doubt not to demolish them fastly.

- Fat loss, you would incline toward not to consume a ton of calories either in light of the fact that it won't be defended, in spite of all the difficulty. A lone cup of stock at the most irksome bit of the fast can help you with overcoming it yet whatever else then that makes you essentially consume more calories right now the weight loss.

- Electrolytes and minerals in bone juices are also mind-boggling for hindering cerebrum fog, lethargy, and evading muscle cramps.

Dry Fasting

- Drinking liquids is furthermore said to have autophagic benefits. One-day of dry fasting is thought to ascend to 3 days of water fasting.

- The idea is that if you deny yourself from water, your body will start to convey its own by changing over the triglycerides from the fat tissue into metabolic water. Hydrogen gets released because of beta-oxidation.

- Fasting has been cleaned in certain exacting and repairing practices. When in doubt, you would incline toward not to get got dried out for a truly significant time-frame. Regardless, consistently time-limited dry fasting of 12-16 hours can be another thing to do if you need further autophagy.

Juice Fasting

- Are furthermore some juice fasting shows where you just drink juices and smoothies. In reality, it could work likewise of the fasting-mimicking diet, yet before long, it's not supported, regardless of any potential benefits.

- Vegetables and normal items make you use a genuine basic proportion of starches and fructose, which will all interfere with both ketosis and autophagy exceptionally hard.

- It can lose a great deal of weight with juice fasting, yet a huge segment of it will be muscle and other fit tissue. That is the explanation you need and ought to be in ketosis to make the fast ensured.

- Or not you're using things like just kale or spinach to make a smoothie, you'd get in all probability log jam the retouching of fasting because of the high proportions of fiber.

- You have to cover hunger or have something to drink that doesn't represent a flavor like water, by then make them stew water with 2 tsp of squeezed apple vinegar. It won't stop the fast and truly has uncommon clinical advantages.

Time-Restricted Feeding

- Feeding created as a thought after the headway of circadian rhythms and chronobiology. Fundamentally, you basically a period limit your step by step food use.

- Supporting has similarly been seemed to thwart metabolic disarranges in mice who have energized a high-fat eating routine without diminishing calories. The mice who have supported their food inside 8 hours didn't get forceful or make infection stood out from the people who ate a comparable proportion of calories with no time impediments. This shows the exhibition of basically time-limiting your food confirmation has huge benefits on general prosperity and body structure. The differentiation may be nearly nothing, yet it's still there.

- The complexity between intermittent fasting and time-confined supporting is that one is done intermittently, for instance, the 36 hour fast while the other should be a bit of your step by step eating plan.

DIFFERENCES BETWEEN THE TYPES OF INTERMITTENT FASTING

The standard similarity is the demonstration of restriction from food and drink. The differentiation, in any case, lies in the point and justification behind fasting-one being for severe and significant reasons, and the other being to shed weight.

Establishments of fasting: A huge amount of what we call 'intermittent fasting' nowadays starts from observational research subject to Ramadan practices and results.

Is an old practice followed in a wide scope of plans by masses comprehensive subject to religion or culture, anyway more starting late in the therapeutic world too for prosperity reasons?

At now, there is actually inadequate evidence for us to perceive what the ideal number of fasting hours should be to propel results.

Of intermittent fasting there are four principal types of intermittent fasting that vary in term and calorie affirmation. These consolidated substitute day is fasting, whole-day fasting, altered fasting frameworks, and time-limited supporting.

Of intermittent fasting are that various people consider it to be an undeniably versatile strategy that doesn't require the specific after of calories, and less orchestrating is required.

Have in like manner showed that intermittent fasting could be as effective for weight loss as a continued with the calorie-limited eating routine.

The 6 Types of Intermittent Fasting to Consider IF

- Of whether you're simply beginning your IF venture or you've had a go at fasting previously, however, couldn't keep it up long haul, this guide will help. Peruse on to discover the seven different types of fasting and which one is directly for your body.

- Are such a significant number of different approaches to do IF, and that is an incredible thing. In the event that this is something you're keen on doing, you can discover the sort that will work best for your way of life, which builds the odds of progress. Here are six:

5:2 Fasting

- It is one of the most well known IF methods. Truth be told, the book The Fast Diet made it standard, and layouts all that you have to think about this methodology. The thought is to eat regularly for five days (don't check calories) and afterward on the other two eat 600 or 600 calories every day for women and men, individually. The fasting days are any days based on your personal preference.

- the thought is that short episodes of fasting keep you agreeable; should you be eager on a fast day, you simply need to anticipate tomorrow when you can "feast" once more. "A few people say 'I can do anything for two days. However, it's a lot to reduce what I eat each of the seven days,'" says Kumar. For these individuals, a 5:2 methodology may work for them over calorie-cutting over the whole week.

- Things considered, the creators of The Fast Diet guidance against making fast days on days where you might be doing a great deal of continuance exercise. In case you're preparing for a bicycle or running race (or run high-mileage weeks), assess if this kind of fasting could work with your preparation plan or talk with a game nutritionist.

Time-Restricted Fasting

- this sort of IF, you pick an eating window consistently, which ought to in a perfect world leave a 14 to 16 hour fast. (Because of hormonal concerns, Women fast for close to 14 hours every day.) "Fasting advances autophagy, the normal 'cell housekeeping' process where the body clears flotsam and jetsam and different things that hold up the traffic of the health of mitochondria, which starts when liver glycogen is exhausted. Doing this may help expand fat cell digestion and enhances insulin work, she says.

- This to work, you may set your eating window from 9 a.m. to 5 p.m., for example. This can work particularly well for somebody with a family who has an early supper, at any rate, says Kumar. At that point, a significant part of the time invested fasting is energy spent dozing in any case. (You additionally don't actually need to "miss" any meals, contingent upon when you set your window.) But this is subject to how steady you can be. On the off chance that your timetable is regularly changing, or you need or need the opportunity to go out to breakfast incidentally, head out for a late-night out on the town, or go to party time, day by day times of fasting may not be for you.

Overnight Fasting

- The methodology is the least difficult of the bundle and includes fasting for a 12-hour time frame each day. For instance: Choose to quit having after supper by 7 p.m. furthermore, continue eating at 7 a.m. with breakfast the following morning. Autophagy does, in any case, occur at the 12-hour mark, however, you'll get progressively mellow cell benefits, . This is the base number of fasting hours she suggests. A genius of this strategy is that it's anything but difficult to actualize. Likewise, you don't need to skip meals; on the off chance that anything, everything you're doing is wiping out asleep time nibble (in the event that you ate one in the first place). This technique doesn't expand the advantages of fasting. In case you're utilizing fasting for weight loss, a little fasting window implies more opportunity to eat, and it may not assist you with diminishing the number of calories you devour.

Entire Day Fasting

- You eat once every day. A few people decide to have supper and afterward not to eat again until the following day's supper, . That implies your fasting period is 24 hours. This varies from the 5:2 technique. Fasting periods are basically 24 hours (supper to supper or lunch to lunch), while at 5:2, the fasting is really 36 hours. (For instance, you have supper on Sunday, "fast" Monday by eating 600 to 600 calories, and break it with breakfast on Tuesday.)

- Bit of leeway is that, whenever accomplished for weight loss, it's extremely intense (however not difficult) to eat a whole day of calories at a time. The detriment to this methodology is that it's difficult to get all the supplements your body needs to work ideally with only one meal. Also, this methodology is hard to adhere to. You may get extremely ravenous when supper moves around, and that can lead you to expend not very good, calorie-thick decisions. Consider it: When you're covetous, you do not actually desire broccoli. Numerous individuals likewise savor espresso abundance to get past their appetite, , which can effectively affect your rest. You may likewise see mind haze for the duration of the day in case you're not eating.

Alternate Day Fasting

- Individuals may take fast every other day, with a fast comprising of 25 percent of their calorie needs (around 600 calories) and nonfasting days being typical eating days. This is a mainstream approach for weight loss. Exchange day fasting was powerful in helping corpulent grown-ups get more fit. The symptoms (like craving) diminished by week two, and the members began feeling progressively fulfilled on a diet after week four. The drawback is that during the two months in the test, members said that they were never truly "full," which can make sticking to this methodology testing.

1. Pick Your-Day Fasting

It is, even more, a pick-your-own experience. You may do the time-confined fasting (fast for 16 hours, eat for eight, for example) each other day or on more than one occasion per week, . This means Sunday may be a typical day of eating, and you'd quit eating by 8 p.m.; at that point, you'd continue eating again on Monday around early afternoon. Basically, it resembles skipping breakfast a couple of days, seven days.

- Show that eating it is related to a lower BMI, yet there's no reliable proof in randomized preliminaries that it will cause weight loss.

- Might be effectively versatile to your way of life and is more take the path of least resistance, which means you can make it work even with a calendar that changes week to week. In any case, looser methodologies may mean progressively gentle benefits.

WHAT TO EAT WHILE DOING INTERMITTENT FASTING

Even diet is the way to getting more fit, keeping up vitality levels and staying with the diet. "Anybody endeavoring to shed pounds should concentrate on supplement thick foods, similar to organic products, veggies, entire grains, nuts, beans, seeds, just as dairy and fit proteins,"

Might you benefit as much as possible from your calorie remittance on a fast day?

High-protein meals, which help you to feel full for more. As protein is genuinely high in calories, you can't have a gigantic sum for your 600 calories; however, make protein your fundamental wellspring of calories.

Off your plate with low-calorie vegetables: they fill your stomach, taste great, and benefit you. Steam them, stove cook with a teaspoon of oil, or pan-fried food and add a few flavors or flavorings to make an extremely scrumptious filling meal. Or then again have them crude in a major plate of mixed greens.

Sugars: they are high in calories and cause you to feel hungry again rapidly. Instances of starch-containing foods to avoid are potatoes, sweet potato, parsnips, rice, pasta, bread, a few organic products (bananas, grapes, melon, prunes, raisins, dates and other dried natural products), breakfast grains, natural product juice, fresh corn/sweetcorn and anything containing sugar, nectar of different syrups.

Not to fear fat: albeit fat is high in calories, it causes you to feel full. Remember limited quantities of fat for your fast day food.

The fact that the prescribed calorie remittance of 600 calories for women; 600 calories for men isn't severe to such an extent that it truly matters on the off chance that you go over or under the stipend by a bit, you should gauge or quantify at any rate the unhealthy fixings in your plans and work out the calorie content.

Is something said about instant meals? An instant meal can be an incredibly simple arrangement. Likewise, with home-prepared meals, search for alternatives that are low in starch and sugar and high in protein and vegetables.

At the end of the day, eat a lot of the underneath foods, and you won't end up in ravenous wrath while fasting.

Water

The fact that you aren't eating, it's critical to remain hydrated for such a huge number of reasons, similar to the health of essentially every significant organ in your body. The measure of water that any one individual should drink shifts; however, you need your pee to be a light yellow shading consistently. Dim yellow pee shows a lack of hydration, which can cause cerebral pains, weariness, and dizziness. Couple that with constrained food, and it could be a catastrophe waiting to happen. In the event that the idea of plain water doesn't energize you, include a crush of the lemon squeeze, a couple of mint leaves, or cucumber cuts to your water. It'll be our little mystery.

Avocado

Might appear to be illogical to eat the most unhealthy organic product while attempting to get more fit; however, the monounsaturated fat in avocado is amazingly satisfying. Including a portion of an avocado to your lunch may keep you full for quite a long time longer than if you didn't eat the green pearl.

Fish

An explanation the Dietary Guidelines proposes eating at any rate eight ounces of fish for every week. In addition to the fact that it is wealthy in healthy fats and protein, it likewise contains plentiful measures of nutrient D. Also, in case you're just eating a constrained measure of food for the duration of the day, don't you need one that conveys increasingly supplement value for your money? Also, that constraining your calorie intake may upset your perception, and fish is frequently viewed as a "mind food."

Cruciferous Veggies

Like broccoli, Brussels sprouts, and cauliflower are, for the most part, loaded with the f-word—fiber. At the point when you're eating inconsistently, it's urgent to eat fiber-rich foods that will keep you customary and forestall blockage. Fiber likewise can cause you to feel full, which is something you may need on the off chance that you can't eat again for 16 hours. Woof.

Potatoes

After me: Not every single white food is terrible. A valid example: Potatoes has been viewed as one of the most satisfying foods around. Eating potatoes as a major aspect of a healthy diet could help with weight loss. Apologies, French fries, and potato chips don't check.

Beans and Legumes

Preferred expansion to stew might be your closest companion on the IF way of life. Food, explicitly carbs, supplies vitality for action. While we're not guiding you to carbo-load, it unquestionably wouldn't damage to toss some low-calorie carbs, similar to beans and vegetables, into your eating plan. Furthermore, foods like chickpeas, dark beans, peas, and lentils have been appeared to diminish body weight, even without calorie limitation.

Probiotics

Know what your gut like the most or crave for? Consistency and assorted variety. That implies they are disturbed when they're eager. Also, when your gut is unsettled, you may encounter some disturbing symptoms, similar to obstruction. To check this disagreeableness, include probiotic-rich foods, like kefir, a fermented tea, or kraut, to your diet. The Farmhouse Culture Gut Shots are ideal for any 600-calorie days since each 1.5-ounce shot is overflowing with live probiotics (10 billion CFUs) for only ten calories.

Berries

Preferred smoothie expansion is ready with crucial supplements. Strawberries are an incredible wellspring of insusceptible boosting nutrient C, with in excess of 100 percent of the everyday esteem in one cup. Furthermore, that is not, in any case, the best part—People who devoured a diet wealthy in flavonoids, similar to those in blueberries and strawberries, had littler increments in BMI over a 14-year time span than the individuals who didn't eat berries.

Eggs

The enormous egg has six grams of protein and concocts in minutes. Getting, however, much protein as could reasonably be expected is significant for keeping full and building muscle. Men who had an egg breakfast rather than a bagel were less eager and ate less for the duration of the day. At the dawn of the day, when you're searching for something to do during your fasting period, why not hard-heat up certain eggs?

Nuts

Might be higher in calories than numerous different bites, yet nuts contain something that most low-quality nourishment doesn't—great fat. Polyunsaturated fat in pecans can really adjust the physiological markers for appetite and satiety.

- More, in case you're stressed over calories, don't be! A one-ounce serving of almonds (around 23 nuts) has 20 percent fewer calories than recorded on the name. Fundamentally, the biting procedure doesn't totally separate the almond cell dividers, leaving a part of the nut unblemished and unabsorbed during processing.

Whole/Entire Grains

- On a tight eating routine and eating carbs appear as though they have a place in two different containers, yet not generally! Entire grains are wealthy in fiber and protein, so eating a little goes far in keeping you full. In addition, eating entire grains rather than refined grains may really fire up your digestion. So feel free to eat your entire grains and adventure out of your customary range of familiarity to attempt farro, bulgur, spelled, Kamut, amaranth, millet, sorghum, or freekeh.

- During intermittent fasting (IF) can be befuddling. This is supposing that isn't a diet plan; however, an eating plan. Remembering this, specialists at Do Fasting have made an intermittent fasting food list that will keep you healthy while you are on your weight loss venture.

- The off chance that informs you concerning when to eat; however, doesn't make reference to what foods can be remembered for your diet. An absence of clear dietary rules can give a bogus impression that one can eat anything they desire. For other people, this can cause issues with picking the "right" foods and beverages.

- Damage your weight-loss endeavors as well as make you bound to be undernourished or overfed.

The Fast Overview of Intermittent-Fasting and Its categories

- Fasting is an inexorably mainstream eating plan. It includes rotating patterns of "sustaining" and "fasting" periods.

- Every one of your calories inside a brief period has been appeared to offer a bunch of health benefits. These incorporate healthy weight loss, improved heart health, and healthy glucose levels. Moreover, IF can likewise help improve emotional wellness and turn around certain impacts of maturing.

Benefits of Intermittent Fasting

To numerous prevailing fashion diets, intermittent fasting is upheld by a solid body of logical proof. This recognise it one of the best devices for healthy weight loss.

There are numerous approaches to do intermittent fasting. Some of them are:

5:2 FAST

Adaptable strategy for fasting is well known among fledglings. Right now, I can eat regularly for five days every week. During the staying 2 days, you should confine your day by day calorie intake to around 600 calories.

12-HOUR FAST

The 5:2 fast, this is another tenderfoot agreeable fasting strategy. It is anything but difficult to follow. Basically, avoid eating any calories for 12 hours. Eat every one of your calories inside the following 12 hours. That finishes one pattern of fasting.

- Your body adjusts to fasting for 12 hours; you can stir your way up to fasting for longer spans, for example, the 16:8 fast or 20-hour fast.

16-HOUR FAST

- Is presumably the most contemplated type of IF. We may state it is an all-inclusive variant of the 12-hour fast. You are not permitted to eat for 16 hours per day and can eat regularly in the 8-hour sustaining window.

20-HOUR FAST OR "THE WARRIOR DIET."

- It is an outrageous type of fasting. It has a long fasting hour/window of 20 hours and a short eating window of 4 hours. The 20-hour fast is undeniably fit for individuals who have invested a lot of energy doing 16-hour fasts.

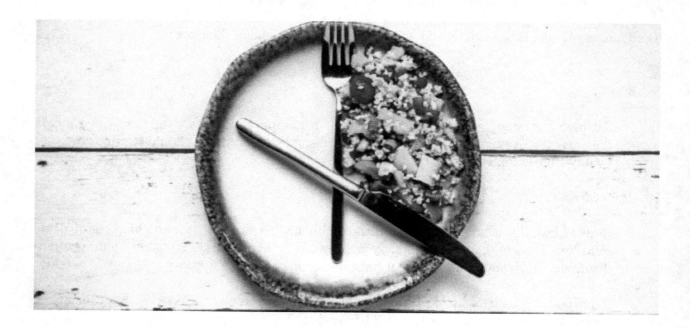

The Intermittent Fasting Food Lists And How to Choose the Best Foods

Intermittent fasting is about being healthy than just fastly losing your weight. Accordingly, it is fundamentally critical to pick supplement thick foods, for example, veggies, organic products, lean proteins, and healthy fats.

intermittent fasting food rundown ought to contain:

FOR PROTEIN

- Recommended Dietary Allowance (RDA) for protein is 0.8 grams of protein per kilogram of body weight. Your necessities may change contingent upon your wellness objectives and level of activity.

- Causes you get in shape by diminishing vitality intake, expanding satiety, and boosting digestion.

- In addition, when joined with quality preparing, expanded protein intake enables work to muscle. Having more muscle in the body normally builds your digestion, as muscle consumes a larger number of calories than fat.

- IF food list for protein includes:

- Poultry and fish

- Eggs

- Seafood

- Dairy items, for example, milk, yogurt, and cheddar.

- Seeds and nuts

- Beans and vegetables

- Soy

- Whole grains

FOR CARBS

- Are the significant wellspring of vitality for your body. The other two are protein and fat. Carbs come in different structures. The most outstanding of them are sugar, fiber, and starch.

- Regularly get negative criticism for causing weight gain. Notwithstanding, not all carbs are made equivalent, and they are not intrinsically stuffing. Whether you will put on weight relies upon the sort and amount of the carbs you eat.

- To pick foods that are high in fiber and starch yet low in sugar.

- Thirty grams of fiber from your diet isn't a tough test. You can get them by eating a basic egg sandwich, Mediterranean grain with chickpeas, apple with nutty spread, and chicken and dark peas enchiladas.

- IF food list for carbs includes:

- Sweet potatoes

- Beetroots

- Quinoa

- Oats

- Brown rice

- Bananas

- Mangoes

- Apples

- Berries

- Kidney beans

- Pears

- Avocado

- Carrots

- Broccoli

- Brussels grows

- Almonds

- Chia seeds

- Chickpeas

FOR FATS

- Ought to contribute 20% to 35% of your day by day calories. Most outstandingly, immersed fat ought not to contribute over 10% of day by day calories.

- It can be acceptable, terrible, or basically in the middle of relying upon the sort.

- Instance, Trans fats increment aggravation, decrease the degrees of the "great" cholesterol and increment the degrees of the "awful" cholesterol. They are found in seared foods and prepared merchandise.

- Fats can expand the danger of heart illness. Be that as it may, master suppositions vary on this. It's insightful to eat them with some restraint. Red meat, entire milk, coconut oil, and heated merchandise contain high measures of immersed fats.

- Fats incorporate monounsaturated and polyunsaturated fats. These fats can decrease the danger of heart sickness, lower circulatory strain, and diminish the blood levels of fats.

- Oil, nut oil, canola oil, safflower oil, sunflower oil, and soybean oils are rich wellsprings of these fats.

- IF food list for fats includes:

- Avocados

- Nuts

- Cheese

- Whole eggs

- Dark chocolate

- Fatty fish

- Chia seeds

- Extra virgin olive oil (EVOO)

- Full-fat yogurt

1. FOR A HEALTHY GUT

- Developing a body of proof shows that your gut health is the way into your overall health. Your gut is home to billions of microscopic organisms known as the smaller scale biota.

- Microscopic organisms influence your gut health, assimilation, and emotional well-being. They may likewise assume a vital job in numerous ceaseless issue.

- In this manner, you should deal with those small bugs in your stomach, particularly when you are intermittent fasting.

- intermittent fasting food list for a healthy gut include:

- All vegetables

- Fermented vegetables

- Kefir

- Kimchi

- Kombucha

- Miso

- Sauerkraut

- Tempeh

- keeping your gut healthy, these foods can likewise assist you with shedding pounds by:

- Decreasing the retention of fat from the gut.

- We are increasing the discharge of ingested fat through stools.

- We are reducing food intake.

1. FOR HYDRATION

- day by day liquid necessity is:

- About 15.5 cups (3.7 liters) for men.

- About 11.5 cups (2.7 liters) for women.

- Incorporate water just like foods and beverages that contain water.

- Hydrated during intermittent fasting is basic to your health. Lack of hydration can cause migraines, outrageous tiredness, and dazedness. On the off chance that you are as of now battling with these symptoms of fasting, lack of hydration can exacerbate them or even genuine.

- intermittent fasting food list for hydration include:

- Water

- Sparkling water

- Black espresso or tea

- Watermelon

- Strawberries

- Cantaloupe

- Peaches

- Oranges

- Skim milk

- Lettuce

- Cucumber

- Celery

- Tomatoes

- Plain yogurt

- Taking a lot of water can likewise help with weight loss. Appropriate hydration can assist you with getting more fit by:

- Decreasing hunger or food intake.

- It is increasing fat consumption.

- to AVOID the Intermittent Fasting Food List

- Processed foods

- Refined grains

- Trans-fat

- Sugar-improved drinks

- Candy bars

- Processed meat

- Alcoholic drinks

THE MYTHS AND MISTAKES

Fasting isn't generally viewed as a diet, yet a specific example of eating. This sort of eating plan has increased enormous notoriety as of late, particularly for women over 60. You may fast for 16 hours and eat during an 8-hour window. This is the 16-8 arrangement and is frequently viewed as the standard. A few people follow each other-day plan with low caloric intake one day and a normal sum the following. The manner in which you take part intermittent fasting to get in shape is famous for an explanation — it works when done effectively.

There are a few potential health benefits when utilizing intermittent fasting. A couple of benefits may incorporate decreased danger of malignant growth, diabetes, and heart infection. It can much trigger autophagy, which is known to help with dementia. Regardless of whether you utilize some of these methods kind of intermittent fasting, it's critical to avoid the traps that can undermine your endeavors. Coming up next are a few intermittent fasting mistakes numerous learners frequently make.

Rolling out Too Many Improvements Too Fastly

You're preparing to begin something new, and you're eager to receive all the rewards as fast as could be expected under the circumstances. It's just characteristic that you need to make a plunge. Be that as it may, attempting to roll out such a large number of improvements too early may disrupt your endeavors.

The key is to begin gradually by including a couple of changes one after another. For instance, if you've chosen to do two 600 calorie days every week while devouring a normal measure of calories the other five, consider beginning with only one 600 calorie day. Following half a month, you can include the second day into your daily schedule.

If you aren't into calorie checking, investigate PLATE, which changes the concentration to divide control.

Not Watching Your Liquid Intake

Staying in a fasting state can be frustrated regardless of whether you're not eating. Most fluids will break the fast and extraordinarily diminish any benefits. Despite the fact that they're fat and sans calorie, it is anything but a smart thought to drink diet soft drinks. Indeed, even sugars that have zero calories can contrarily influence your insulin levels.

The essential fluid you ought to drink during your fast is water. A moderate measure of espresso won't break your fast. You'll need to take your espresso dark, in any case. Indeed, even a little sugar in your espresso or lemon in your water can influence the fasting time frame.

Not Drinking Enough Water

While it's significant not to drink inappropriate fluids when fasting, it's similarly as essential to ensure you drink enough water. Not getting enough water can make you hungry, and it's anything but difficult to some of the time mistake long for thirst.

Individuals get a great deal of water from a considerable lot of the foods they eat. Worldwide Food Information expresses that 20 percent of the water our bodies use originates from food. This implies in case you're not eating for a few hours; you'll have to drink around 20 percent more water than expected to compensate for any shortfall.

Eating Unhealthy Foods

Since intermittent fasting isn't generally a diet plan, there aren't any foods that are untouchable. This can lead numerous individuals to fall into the snare of topping off on lousy nourishment or making a beeline for the inexpensive food drive-through the moment their fast is up. Try not to make a propensity for eating unhealthy on the grounds that you think fasting compensates for it.

Cause a rundown of all the healthy foods you to appreciate. Do ordinary shopping for food and remain composed with regards to your food decisions. While fulfilling a hankering with not exactly healthy snacks sometimes is alright, for ideal health and weight-loss achievement, it's important to eat as healthy as could be expected under the circumstances. Eating the correct foods is vital to taking advantage of any weight loss plan. Foods wealthy in calcium, protein, and B-12 ought to be high on the rundown, particularly for women over 60.

Overeating After Each Fast

This is presumably the greatest trap for the two amateurs just as the individuals who have been fasting intermittently for quite a while. Utilizing intermittent fasting to get more fit will reverse discharge in the event that you expend such a large number of calories during an opportunity to eat.

One approach to shield from overeating is to devour larger amounts of healthier foods during your eating window. This would incorporate heaps of healthy plates of mixed greens and crisp vegetables. It's additionally a smart thought to be set up by arranging meals and having fixings prepared before your fast closures. Thusly you're not enticed to simply snatch anything. Remember that it can take as long as about fourteen days until you've changed in accordance with the point that you won't feel as eager after each fasting period.

Attempting to Stick to the Wrong Plan

There are loads of different approaches to join intermittent fasting into your daily schedule. For instance, if your fasting plan incorporates not eating from 8 pm until early afternoon every day and you have an upsetting activity that begins promptly in the first part of the day, this is most likely not the correct arrangement for you.

What works for one individual, may not fill in as viably for another person. To receive the most rewards of intermittent fasting, you have to analyze a piece with different types of plans. It's alright on the off chance that it takes a little while or longer to locate the correct arrangement that works for you.

Practicing Too Much or Too Little

It's imperative to remain genuinely dynamic. If you would prefer not to overdo it, particularly when you're fasting. A few novices may feel overwhelmed, beginning another eating technique, and may overlook exercise altogether. Others might be eager to such an extent that they overdo it.

It's a smart thought to pick a moderate exercise schedule, particularly when beginning. Strolling the pooch for twenty minutes or riding your bicycle to work are simple approaches to add moderate exercise to your customary calendar.

In case you're keen on working intermittent fasting into your weight the board plan, PLATE is an incredible asset. It utilizes intermittent fasting to get more fit and is made particularly for women over 60. PLATE assists women with coming to and keep up healthy weight objectives by concentrating on parcel control and responsibility from other women.

1-Not Drinking Enough Water

Maybe one of the most squeezing and effectively avoidable intermittent fasting mistakes isn't taking in enough water.

We realize drinking water is significant for overall health, obviously, yet it's extra significant when you're fasting.

Why? Since a significant part of when we believe we're eager, we're really parched.

Would you be able to envision how your craving might be influenced in case you're one of them while attempting to go the main part of the day without eating?

Fortunately, this is very simple to avoid!

Sneaking more water into your day is as simple as making a couple of basic changes.

A few people truly get exhausted by drinking plain water. Trust me, one thing that is a great idea to do is to add a couple of Mio Drops to water, and it will have a tremendous effect!

In the event that you don't think about these, Mio Drops are zero-calorie, zero-carb, without sugar water enhancers that arrive in a minor squirt bottle.

You simply press two or three drops into your water, and you're all set!

The Fruit Punch is the best one, IMO,

2-Doing Too Much, Too Soon

3-Adding Artificial Sweetener during Fasting Windows

4-Misunderstanding Real Hunger Cues

Perhaps the best thing that I've taken from my intermittent fasting test is that I found a good pace genuine appetite is.

It doesn't come at 9 am when you've been wakeful for 60 minutes, and last ate a late-night nibble at 11 pm the prior night.

Like no doubt, your stomach may be snarling.

You may have a desire for something yummy.

It may be wonderful to plunk down with your family or companions and appreciate the social part of feasting.

Yet, you aren't generally eager.

Intermittent fasting instructs you that on the off chance that you stand by sufficiently long (and normally only 5 to 10 minutes), more often than not, your "hunger" will blur.

It's most likely transpired ordinarily before without you in any event, thinking about it.

How frequently at work have you intended to go eat; however, some squeezing business-related undertaking came up, and an hour or two passed by, and you'd overlooked your once protesting stomach?

At the point when you're extremely ravenous, you won't forget about it.

In any case, yielding and eating too early is one of the serious mix-ups with intermittent fasting. Supposing that you simply drink some water and allow it 10 minutes or somewhere in the vicinity, you'll, as a rule, be okay.

Try not to crash your intermittent fasting plan before you even begin.

Try not to tragically give in to bogus craving!

5-Using Intermittent Fasting As an Excuse to Overeat

One of the most hostile intermittent fasting mistakes is embracing the disposition that says, "I've starved myself throughout the day, I DESERVE to remunerate myself for supper"!

At that point, go take off with a crazy measure of unhealthy, calorie bombarding garbage.

Try not to be that young lady.

You'll feel hopeless AND most likely put on weight.

Absolutely not cool.

In spite of the fact that actually, intermittent fasting isn't a diet in that it doesn't confine what you eat, it's as yet critical to settle on food decisions that are on the healthier side.

You can totally overeat and put on weight by eating just once per day in case you're eating a greater number of calories than your body consumes.

While you don't need to be an absolute stickler and there's space for adaptability, be shrewd.

Help yourself out and don't go crazy during your encouraging window.

6-Not Eating Enough

On the other side, on the off chance that you've yet to attempt intermittent fasting before, this may appear to be illogical.

In any case, for some fasters, when you don't eat for an all-inclusive timeframe, you really become less ravenous.

I believe that is the reason I had the option to fast 24 hours my first day.

Furthermore, why on the off chance that you glance around (like in Reddit's r/fasting discussion), you'll see individuals doing truly cracking overly long fasts like a month and such.

Fasting can thoroughly murder your appetite.

Except if you're deliberately doing an all-encompassing fast (not suggested for fledglings), however, it's extremely simple to do as such, it is anything but a smart thought to under-eat either.

On the off chance that you under eat sufficiently long, you can absolutely wreck your digestion and toss your hormones crooked.

Moreover, you'll deny your body of fundamental supplements, which can prompt health gives that are far more terrible than conveying a couple of additional pounds.

Counsel with your primary care physician about a sheltered, healthy calorie extend for weight loss and ensure you're someplace around that run most days for ideal outcomes.

7-Failing to Plan Your Meals In Advance

While calorie tallying isn't important (however truly, you'll show signs of improvement results on the off chance that you do it), having a harsh thought of how you'll break your fast is an unbelievable intermittent fasting hack.

By postponing when you eat, you're permitting yourself an opportunity to be less indiscreet.

Rather than going "I'm STARVING and need to eat NOW," at that point swerving into the closest cheap food drive-through path to execute that hunger ASAP, you're learning "meh… I feel hungry, yet I can pause".

Utilizing this opportunity to consider what you'll eat when you eat, and settling on healthier decisions just causes you over the long haul.

It shows you how to eat for fruitful weight loss, while decreasing caloric intake, keeping you sustained, and boosting your certainty.

In case you're fasting for 16 hours, you can take as meager as 5 minutes to arrange for how you'll break that fast later.

It's truly not unreasonably hard and will prepare for a slimmer future!

8-Not Exercising At All

While it's actually you could, in any case, lose a lot of intermittent weight fasting in the event that you never worked out, for what reason would you pass up the mind-blowing chance to lose significantly increasingly, faster?

It truly has neither rhyme nor reason.

Time will be time. A month is a month.

In the event that in one month you could be languid and shed 5 pounds or exercise three times each week and lose 10, wouldn't you lean toward the ten?

9-Failing to Develop Healthy Eating Habits for The Long Haul

10-Telling Too Many People you're Intermittent Fasting

11-Choosing the Wrong Program

12-Giving Up Too Soon

SOME NUTRITIONAL FACTS (NOT TOO SCIENCE)

The Facts About Intermittent Fasting, Fat Loss, And Muscle Growth

Defenders of intermittent fasting put forth a convincing defense for their methodology. Be that as it may, is it best for your objectives?

In the wellness business, something other than about any industry that rings a bell, limits are the standard. What is the state of affairs today will be trash tomorrow, and the contrary will turn into business as usual? I discussed this in my digital book "The Science of Sugar and Fat-Loss," however it applies to lifts and practices just as supplements.

Consider it: 10 years back, bodybuilders evaded the enormous lifts of squat, seat, and deadlift. Presently it appears as though every self-important bodybuilder is utilizing a DUP format for squat, seat, and deadlift. Not excessively, there's an issue with that approach; I'm a fanatic of the huge three lifts.

Eating plans are certainly dependent upon these epic emotional episodes too. Ten years back, bodybuilder rationale had everybody in the exercise center, eating every 2-3 hours to "stir the metabolic fire" and remain anabolic. Today, the exercise center is excited to talk about not eating for up to 16-20 hours in a row, what is known as "intermittent fasting."

Both of the listed have their diehard followers, and I'm not here to state that one is in every case right or the other dead off-base. Be that as it may, we should explore the rationale behind both so we can make sense of what will work best for you.

The Old Way: Eat, Eat, Eat

We should start by taking a gander at the old "eat every 2-3 hours" technique, and specifically its cases about metabolic rate first. It has been proposed by innumerable specialists over the years that eating all the more much of the time will improve overall metabolic rate. While I'll concede that the rationale at first sounds great, it doesn't appear to stand the litmus trial of the logical proof.

Practically every examination analyzing meal recurrence in an ongoing meta-investigation exhibited zero contrasts in fat loss when calories were controlled. Shockingly, there additionally don't seem, by all accounts, to be contrasted in markers of cravings with changes in meal recurrence, and metabolic rate was not influenced by meal recurrence.

This may appear to be godless to the sincere adherents of the 6-8-meals-per-day mantra, yet it's hard to contend with the information. In any case, it's important this is with respect to fat loss. At the point when quality and muscle gains are the objectives, three full dinners daily may not give enough protein dispersion.

That is the reason, in my PH3 Power and Hypertrophy program, I advocate 4-5 protein-rich meals every day, contingent upon your own inclination. Any less and you will be left packing insane measures of protein into singular meals, which, as I'll talk about somewhat later, likewise is certainly not a smart thought.

The New Way: Fast, Then Feast

So if eight meals are off the table, it naturally implies you ought to do intermittent fasting, right? The most significant factor for long haul achievement in dieting isn't the point at which you eat; it's adherence. It's hard to believe, but it's true: People don't bomb diets since they don't have the ideal meal recurrence, food sources, or supernatural voodoo purify; they bomb diets since they just can't adhere to them.

Individuals who lose a lot of weight, most of them will recover the weight they initially lost, and following five years, they regularly surpass their underlying weight.

This is an enormous issue, and to tackle it, the emphasis ought to be on using methodologies that improve dietary adherence.

Along these lines, if intermittent fasting permits an individual to more readily fit a diet into their way of life and adhere to that diet that is a sufficient contention for me— in any event as to that individual. I've known numerous individuals who had the option to certain fast pieces of the day because of the absence of appetite at those occasions, or essentially in light of the fact that they had exceptionally bustling employments and that way of eating fit their way of life better.

There's another bit of leeway, obviously. Spread, say, 2,600 calories over 6-8 meals, and you'll wind up with some quite unimportant bits. However, those equivalent calories over 1-2 meals can make for a phenomenal food festivity. Numerous individuals like to hold out somewhat longer to have bigger meals. I realize that when I dropped from eight meals for each day to four meals for each day, I was considerably more fulfilled, and my appetite levels dropped.
Would you be able to take this excessively far? Obviously. Numerous individuals discover they basically can't go 12 hours or more without getting greedily ravenous, and this may make them bound to the gorge. For others with confused eating propensities, they may begin getting free with their nourishing windows or accumulating food.

This is what I mean: An ordinary intermittent-fasting convention is regularly 16 hours fasting with 8 hours nourishing, plus or minus a couple of hours. However, a few people will slide into, state, 22/2, and I've even observed individuals go days without eating so as to legitimize and tremendous gorge. That isn't a flaw of intermittent fasting itself, yet it unquestionably implies that it's anything but a suitable convention for everybody. Along these lines, understanding your inclinations toward food and what you like is critical.

So if you lean toward fasting, and it causes you to be progressively disciple to a diet, at that point by all methods do it. In any case, remember that it's not enchantment, and it tends to be fouled up. Fat loss is eventually an issue of calories, not timekeepers.

A Modified Fast for Max Muscle Growth

It's turning out to be certain that while your day by day protein intake is significant, so is the amount you expend per meal and how those meals are conveyed. Be that as it may, while a great many people utilize this acknowledgment just to contend for more protein per meal, there might be a point of consistent losses that is significant for intermittent fasters to consider.

With regards to upgrading muscle protein blend, over expending protein at once of the day couldn't compensate for low protein at some other point of the day. So similarly as there is a characterized protein edge to start anabolism, there likewise has all the earmarks of being a maximal anabolic top. In real life, this implies on the off chance that you just eat a modest quantity of protein a large portion of the day, yet then you eat a huge amount of protein at one meal, it won't "balance out."

For instance, how about we imagine that this anabolic top is 40 grams protein, and the base protein required to start anabolism is 15 grams—this is all hypothetical, all things considered. Clearly, you wouldn't be anabolic during your 16-hour fast. In any case, at that point, to get your 200 grams of protein in that eight-hour window at three meals, you could be expending around 65 grams of protein at every meal. This is just about 60 percent over the hypothetical anabolic top.

For the regular person simply hoping to lean up, this may not be a serious deal. In the event that you need a portion of the benefits from intermittent fasting, however, need to streamline bulk, I would educate a different sort with respect to fast. As opposed to removing all calories, basically, confine carbs and fats during your fasting window, yet keep on equitably disperse your protein intake for the duration of the day. Until we realize where this conceivable anabolic top is, this strikes me as more successful than attempting to pack everything into your nourishing "window."

Adopt this strategy, and you are as yet going to get a huge volume of food in the bolstering time frame and spend a huge bit of the day in a low-insulin fat-consuming state, yet you'll have the option to disperse protein, so that is better for muscle development.

HOW TO FIND THE BEST METHOD OF IF FOR YOU (BASED ON YOUR BODY TYPE, WEIGHT, LIFESTYLE, USUAL STUFF)

Intermittent fasting is notable, yet it's just a hint of something larger with regards to fasting diets all in all. There are for all intents and purposes boundless ways you can embrace a fasting system that suits your own way of life and health needs. We should investigate all the different fasting diets, the health benefits they may bring, and how to do them securely.

Intermittent Fasting (IF) is the willful swearing off food for a predefined period, as a rule around 16 hours with a window of 8 hours to expend meals. Most generally, this is accomplished by skipping breakfast and having the primary meal of the day at around early afternoon, yet a few people interpret intermittent as meaning restraint of somewhere in the range of 12 to 18 hours.

If you have been following a daily practice of intermittent fasting for quite a while and have been an enthusiastic admirer of this propensity, then it is difficult to leave this propensity when you are pregnant. Be that as it may, in the event that you are truly anticipating an infant, you have to change your propensity. You have to follow an increasingly customary calendar.

While following intermittent fasting, you should have regularly skipped breakfast or not taken anything after supper. While this can be an incredible method to get thinner, it very well may be a perilous practice to follow when you are pregnant. Specialists who work in cardiology, weight loss, and sustenance do weight on the point that intermittent fasting may have a job in checking aggravation, cell adjustment, boosting cell adjustment, and streamlining vitality digestion.

Impact of Intermittent Fasting on Pregnant Women

Benefits of intermittent fasting might be far lesser contrasted with the dangers for a pregnant lady. A look at the differed structures of intermittent fasting is as per the following.

- Once seven days you have to fast for 24 hours at a stretch.

- Fast for 16 hours at a solitary go and in the staying 8 hours, crunch in as a lot of calories as you can.

- The impact of intermittent fasting on pregnant women isn't indisputable enough. Be that as it may, specialists don't typically suggest fasting during pregnancy as a result of the accompanying reasons.

- Doctors and dieticians contend that intermittent fasting can trigger unpredictable monthly cycles, nervousness, and restlessness in women. This is clearly not a decent condition for anybody, not to mention a pregnant lady.

- It is accepted that the body has a characteristic inclination of setting off a pressure reaction when you are denied food. This reaction might be minor in men, however significant in women, which might be taken as a sign that the framework wouldn't like to support a child under such conditions.

- Animal contemplates demonstrated that guys of the species can adapt to fasting in a better manner looked at than females. This can be measured from the genuinely steady degrees of male hormones just as intellectual limit subsequent to fasting.

- Females of similar species have given clear indications of diminished richness alongside the significant pressure reaction. Indeed, even the menstrual cycles likewise become deregulated. Notwithstanding, to get the genuine picture, you have to experience a few examinations on fasting during pregnancy.

Impacts of fasting in pregnancy

The impact of fasting on pregnant women is unquestionably deceptive, yet have taken the assistance of strict and conventional practices, and concentrated the impact of these practices on pregnant women of those religions and spots.

A few investigations were led on the pregnant women taking to fasting to watch the sacred month of Ramadan in Islamic societies. It was seen that fasting had a heading on the example just as recurrence of breathing of the hatchling.

Another investigation in 2014 has discovered that it might bring about the lower weight of the infant during childbirth. This is absolutely something to be worried about. Nonetheless, there is another view as well, which expresses that the accessibility of copious food may offer ascent to gestational diabetes. It might likewise bring about high birth weights for babies. Fasting during pregnancy doesn't appear to have an unfavorable impact. The result right now measured on the serum lipid levels of the pregnant lady, the development of blood through the umbilical corridor, and some different elements. Be that as it may, the women tried on this event were all healthy women.

Intermittent Fasting Explained

Regularly alluded to as time-limited sustaining, intermittent fasting is a trick all term for diets which center around going through a piece of the day without eating (fasting), trailed by a timeframe in which you do then expend food.

65

Similarly, as everybody is a person, there is nobody size-fits-all methodology with regards to intermittent fasting.

Actually, there are a wide range of styles of IF that you can pick dependent on your present timetable and wants:

Hormones That Promote Fat Burning

During times of fasting, the body, despite everything, expects vitality to work.

This vitality can emerge out of different sources, for example, glycogen (put away glucose) from the muscle and liver, or it can emerge out of fat.

At the point when you fast, and blood glucose drops low, this powers the emission of a hormone from the pancreas called glucagon.

At the point when glucagon levels rise, this starts a procedure called gluconeogenesis in which the body changes over glucose from non-starchy sources, for example, protein, or discharges glucose from the liver.

On the other hand, this expansion in glucagon can start a procedure of using fat for vitality, one of the principle benefits of intermittent fasting.

Strikingly, fasting likewise expands levels of hormones called catecholamines.

These catecholamine hormones can join to receptors situated on the films of fat cells. When appended, unsaturated fats put away in these cells are discharged into course, to eventually meet their destiny of being oxidized, or "copied."

This procedure of discharging unsaturated fats into the blood is called lipolysis and examines show that intermittent fasting is particularly proficient at actuating it.

Together, this expansion in glucagon and lipolysis is an ideal blend for expanding the measure of weight that is lost specifically from fat tissue.

Approaches to Loosing Weight with Intermittent Fasting

There are a lot range of approaches to get more fit.

One that has gotten famous as of late is called intermittent fasting.

This is a method for eating that includes ordinary momentary fasts.

Fasting for brief periods assists individuals with eating fewer calories and furthermore enhances a few hormones identified with weight control.

There are a few different intermittent fasting methods. Three mainstream ones are:

1. **The 16/8 Method:** Skip breakfast each day and eat during an 8-hour sustaining window, for example, from 12 early afternoons to 8 pm.

2. **Eat-Stop-Eat:** Do a couple of 24-hour fasts every week, for instance, by not having from supper one day until supper the following day.

3. **The 5:2 Diet:** Eating 600-600 calories on two days of the week, however, eat regularly the other 5 days.

For whatever length of time that you don't repay by eating substantially more during the non-fasting periods, at that point, these methods will prompt diminished calorie intake and assist you with getting thinner and midsection fat.

How Intermittent Fasting Affects Your Hormones

Body fat is the body's method for putting away vitality (calories).

At the point when we don't eat anything, the body changes a few things to make the put-away vitality progressively available.

This has to do with changes in sensory system action, just as a significant change in a few essential hormones.

Here is a portion of the things that adjustment in your digestion when you fast:

- **Insulin:** Insulin increments when we eat. At the point when we fast, insulin diminishes drastically. Lower levels of insulin encourage fat consumption.

- **Human development hormone (HGH):** Levels of development hormone may soar during a fast, expanding as much as 5-overlay. The development hormone is a hormone that can help fat loss and muscle gain, in addition to other things.

- **Norepinephrine (noradrenaline):** The sensory system sends norepinephrine to the fat cells, making them separate body fat into free unsaturated fats that can be singed for vitality.

Strikingly, in spite of what the 5-6 meals everyday advocates would have you accept, momentary fasting may really build fat consumption.

Fasting for around 48 hours helps digestion by 3.6-14%. In any case, fasting periods that are longer can smother digestion.

Transient fasting prompts a few changes in the body that make fat-consuming simpler. This incorporates diminished insulin, expanded development hormone, improved epinephrine flagging, and a little lift indigestion.

How Intermittent Fasting Helps to Reduce Calories and Lose Weight.

The primary explanation that intermittent fasting works for weight loss is that it causes you to eat fewer calories.

The entirety of the different conventions includes skipping meals during fasting time frames. Except if you repay by eating significantly more during the eating time frames, at that point, you will be taking in fewer calories.

Intermittent fasting can prompt noteworthy weight loss. Right now, fasting was found to decrease body weight by 3-8% over a time of 3-24 weeks.

While looking at the pace of weight loss, individuals lost about 0.55 pounds (0.25 kg) every week with intermittent fasting. However, 1.65 pounds (0.75 kg) every week with substitute day fasting.

Individuals additionally lost 4-7% of their abdomen boundary, demonstrating that they lost midsection fat.

These outcomes are exceptionally great, and they do show that intermittent fasting can be a valuable weight loss help.

All that being stated, the benefits of intermittent fasting go route past simply weight loss. It additionally has various benefits for metabolic health, and may even assistance forestall incessant ailment and growing life expectancy.

In spite of the fact that calorie checking is commonly not required while doing intermittent fasting, the weight loss is, for the most part, interceded by an overall decrease in calorie intake.

Intermittent fasting and ceaseless calorie limitation show no distinction in weight loss if calories are coordinated between gatherings.

Intermittent fasting is an advantageous method to limit calories without intentionally attempting to eat less. Numerous examinations show that it can assist you with getting in shape and gut fat.

The Intermittent Fasting Helps To Hold on to Muscle When Dieting

One of the most exceedingly terrible symptoms of dieting is that the body will, in general, consume muscle just as fat.

Strikingly, there are a few examinations demonstrating that intermittent fasting might be useful for clutching muscle while losing body fat.

In one survey study, intermittent calorie limitation caused a comparative measure of weight loss as nonstop calorie limitation, yet with a lot littler decrease in bulk.

In the calorie, limitation considers, 25% of the weight loss was bulk, contrasted with just 10% in the intermittent calorie limitation contemplates.

In any case, there were a few confinements to these examinations, so think about the discoveries while taking other factors into consideration.

There is some proof that intermittent fasting can assist you with clutching more bulk when dieting, contrasted with standard calorie limitation.

Intermittent Fasting Makes Healthy Eating Simpler

As I would like to think, one of the fundamental benefits of intermittent fasting is its effortlessness.

I, for one, do the 16/8 technique, where I just eat during a specific "bolstering window" every day.

Rather than eating 3+ meals every day, I eat just 2, which makes it significantly simpler and less complex to keep up my healthy way of life.

The best "diet" for you to hold on to is the one you can adhere to over the long haul. If intermittent fasting makes it simpler for you to adhere to a healthy diet, at that point, this has evident benefits for long haul health and weight support.

One of the principal benefits of intermittent fasting is that it makes healthy eating less complex. This may make it simpler to adhere to a healthy diet over the long haul.

The most effective method to Succeed With an Intermittent Fasting Protocol

There are a few things you have to remember whether you need to shed pounds with intermittent fasting:

1. Food quality: The foods you eat are as yet significant. Attempt to eat for the most part entire, single fixing foods.

2. Calories: Calories despite everything check. Attempt to eat "typically" during the non-fasting periods, less that you make up for the calories you missed by fasting.

3. Consistency: Same similarly as with some other weight loss strategy, you have to stay with it for an all-inclusive timeframe in the event that you need it to work.

4. Patience: It can take as much time as is needed to adjust to an intermittent fasting convention. Attempt to be predictable with your meal calendar, and it will get simpler.

The greater part of the famous intermittent fasting conventions additionally prescribes quality preparing. This is significant on the off chance that you need to consume generally body fat while clutching muscle.

At the outset, calorie tallying is commonly not required with intermittent fasting. If your weight loss slows down, at that point, calorie tallying can be a valuable apparatus.

With intermittent fasting, you, despite everything, need to eat healthily and keep up a calorie shortage on the off chance that you need to get in shape. Being reliable is completely critical, and quality preparation is significant.

WHEN YOU CAN COMBINE IF WITH OTHER DIETS (LIKE KETO, DASH, MEDITERRANEAN, VEGAN OR VEGETARIAN) AND HOW TO DO IT, AND WHEN YOU BETTER DON'T AND WHY

Food joining is a way of thinking of eating that has antiquated roots. However, it has gotten amazingly famous in the ongoing past.

Defenders of food-joining diets accept that ill-advised food blends can prompt sickness, poison development, and stomach related misery.

They additionally accept that legitimate mixes can soothe these issues.

However, is there any fact to these cases?

Food joining is the term for the possibility that specific foods pair well together, while others don't.

The conviction is that joining foods inappropriately — for instance, eating steak with potatoes — can prompt negative health and stomach related impacts.

Food consolidating standards initially showed up in the Ayurvedic medication of antiquated India. However, they turned out to be all the more broadly advanced in the mid-1800s under the term trophology, or "the study of food joining."

The standards of food joining were resuscitated in the mid-1900s by the Hay diet. From that point forward, they've become an establishment for some advanced diets.

For the most part, food-consolidating diets dole out foods to different gatherings.

These are typically separated into carbs and starches, natural products (counting sweet organic products, acidic leafy foods), vegetables, proteins, and fats.

On the other hand, a few plans order foods as either acidic, basic, or unbiased.

Food-consolidating diets indicate how you should join these gatherings in a meal.

Model Rules of Food Combining

The laws of food consolidating can change fairly relying upon the source, yet the most widely recognized standards incorporate the accompanying:

- Only eat natural products on an unfilled stomach, particularly melons.

- Don't join starches and proteins.

- Don't join starches with acidic foods.

- Don't join different types of protein.

- Only expend dairy items on a vacant stomach, particularly milk.

Different guidelines incorporate that protein ought not to be blended in with fat, sugar should just be eaten alone, and products of the soil ought to be eaten independently.

Two Beliefs behind Food Combining

The standards of food consolidating are, for the most part, dependent on two convictions.

The first is that on the grounds that different foods are processed at different rates, consolidating a fast processing food with a moderate processing food causes a "car influx" in your stomach related tract, prompting negative stomach related and health outcomes.

The subsequent conviction is that different foods require different proteins to be separated and that these catalysts work at different pH levels — levels of sharpness — in your gut.

The thought is that if two foods require different pH levels, the body can't appropriately process both simultaneously.

Defenders of food-joining diets accept that these standards are fundamental to legitimate health and processing.

It is additionally accepted that the inappropriate mix of foods prompts negative health results, for example, stomach related misery, the creation of poisons, and illness.

Food consolidating alludes to a method for eating wherein specific types of foods are not eaten together. Defenders of food-consolidating diets accept inappropriate mixes that lead to illness and stomach related trouble.
Up until this point, just one examination has analyzed the standards of food join. It tried whether a diet-dependent on food was consolidating affected weight loss.

Members were part into two gatherings and given either a fair diet or a diet-dependent on the standards of food consolidating.

On the two diets, they were just permitted to eat 1,100 calories for each day.

Following a month and a half, members in the two gatherings had lost a normal of around 13–18 lbs (6–8 kg), however, the food-joining diet offered no advantage over the decent diet.

Truth be told, there is no proof to help the vast majority of the as far as anyone knows logical standards of food consolidating.

Huge numbers of the first food-joining diets were grown over 100 years back when significantly less was thought about human nourishment and assimilation.

Yet, what is presently thought about essential organic chemistry and nutritional science legitimately repudiates the vast majority of the standards of food join.

Here's a more intensive guide to take at the science behind the cases.

On Avoiding Mixed Meals

The expression "blended meals" alludes to meals that contain a mix of fat, carbs, and protein.

The guidelines of food joining are, to a great extent, dependent on the possibility that the body isn't prepared to process blended meals.

Be that as it may, this is essentially not the situation. The human body developed on a tight eating routine of entire foods, which quite often contain a mix of carbs, protein, and fat.

For instance, vegetables and grains are normally viewed as carb-containing foods. Be that as it may, they all additionally contain a few grams of protein for every serving. Also, meat is viewed as protein food, yet even lean meat contains some fat.

In this way — in light of the fact that numerous foods contain a mix of carbs, fat, and protein — your stomach related tract is constantly arranged to process a blended meal.

At the point when food enters your stomach, gastric corrosive is discharged. The chemicals pepsin and lipase are likewise discharged, which help start protein and fat assimilation.

Intermittent fasting and the keto diet

With regards to biohacking, there most likely aren't two more famous practices than the ketogenic high-fat diet and fasting.

The two regimens have health benefits, including improved digestion, weight loss, and far better subjective capacity. Research reads have demonstrated benefits for each, and individual stories via web-based networking media fill in as some truly significant tales.

Ketosis is the way toward consuming ketone bodies for vitality.

On an ordinary diet, your body consumes glucose as its essential fuel source. Overabundance glucose is put away as glycogen. At the point when your body is denied of glucose (because of exercise, intermittent fasting, or a ketogenic diet), it will go to glycogen for vitality. Simply after glycogen is exhausted, will your body begin consuming fat.

A ketogenic diet, which is also called a low-carb, high-fat diet, makes a metabolic move that permits your body to separate fat into ketone bodies in the liver for vitality. There are three fundamental ketone bodies found in your blood, pee, and breath:

- **Acetoacetate:** The primary ketone to be made. It can either be changed over into beta-hydroxybutyrate or transformed into CH3)2CO.

- **Acetone:** Created precipitously from the breakdown of acetoacetate. It's the most unpredictable ketone and is frequently perceptible in the breath when somebody initially goes into ketosis.

- **Beta-hydroxybutyrate (BHB):** This is the ketone that is utilized for vitality and the richest in your blood once you're completely in ketosis. It's additionally the sort found in exogenous ketones and what ketogenic blood tests measure.

Intermittent Fasting and Its Relation to Ketosis

Intermittent fasting comprises of eating just inside a particular timeframe and not eating for the rest of the hours of the day. Each individual, regardless of whether they're mindful of it or not, fasts overnight from supper to breakfast.

The benefits of fasting have been utilized for a huge number of years in Ayurveda and Traditional Chinese Medicine as an approach to help reset your digestion and help your gastrointestinal framework subsequent to overeating.

There are numerous ways to deal with intermittent fasting, with different time periods:

- 16-20 hours fasting period

- Alternate-day fasting

- 24-hour day fasting

If you need to begin fasting, one well-known rendition is the 16/8 keto intermittent fasting technique, where you eat inside an 8-hour eating window (for instance, 11 a.m. to 7 p.m.), trailed by a 16-hour fasting window.

Other fasting plans incorporate the 20/4 or 14/10 methods, while a few people incline toward doing an entire 24-hour fasting day on more than one occasion for each week.

Intermittent fasting can place you in a condition of ketosis faster in light of the fact that your cells will rapidly expand your glycogen stores, and afterward begin utilizing your put away fat for fuel. This prompts a fastening of the fat-consuming procedure and expanded ketone levels.

Ketosis versus intermittent Fasting: The Physical Benefits

Both the ketogenic diet and the intermittent fasting can be compelling instruments for:

- Healthy weight loss

- Fat loss, not muscle loss

- Balancing cholesterol levels

- Improving insulin affectability

- Keeping glucose levels stable.

Ketogenic diet for Weight Loss, Fat Loss, and Improved Cholesterol.

The keto diet radically diminishes your carb intake, compelling your body to consume fat as opposed to glucose. This makes it a successful apparatus for weight loss, yet in addition to the administration of diabetes, insulin obstruction, and even heart infection.

While singular outcomes shift, keto has reliably prompted a decrease in weight and body fat rate in a wide scope of circumstances.

Members who followed a low-sugar keto meal plan essentially diminished body weight, body fat rate, and fat mass, losing a normal of 7.6 pounds and 2.6% body fat while keeping up fit bulk.

Watching the long haul impacts of a keto diet in hefty individuals found that their weight and body mass diminished drastically over the course of two years. The individuals who definitely diminished their sugar intake saw a critical decline in LDL (awful) cholesterol, triglycerides, and improved insulin affectability.

They have contrasted a ketogenic diet with eating fewer calories in hefty youngsters and grown-ups. The outcomes indicated kids following the keto diet lost more body weight, fat mass, and all-out midriff boundary altogether. They likewise demonstrated an emotional decline in the insulin levels, the biomarker of type 2 diabetes.

Fat Loss for Intermittent Fasting and Maintaining Muscle Mass

Intermittent fasting can be a proficient weight loss instrument, some of the time being significantly more helpful than just limiting your calorie intake.
In one examination, intermittent fasting was demonstrated to be as compelling as ceaseless calorie limitation in battling heftiness. In examines done by the NIH, weight loss was accounted for over 84% of the members — regardless of which fasting plan they picked

Like ketosis, intermittent fasting can advance fat loss while keeping up fit bulk. In one examination, scientists inferred that individuals who fasted would do well to weight loss results (while safeguarding muscle) than the individuals who followed a low-calorie diet, despite the fact that the all-out caloric intake was the equivalent.

Ketosis versus Intermittent Fasting: Mental Benefits

Past their physiological benefits, both intermittent fasting and ketosis give different mental benefits. Both have been experimentally appeared to

- Boost memory

- Improve mental clearness and core interest

- Prevent neurological maladies including Alzheimer's and epilepsy

Keto for Improving Brain Fog and Memory

On a carb-based diet, the vacillations in your glucose levels can cause changes in vitality levels — these are known as sugar rushes and sugar crashes. In ketosis, your cerebrum utilizes a progressively steady wellspring of fuel: ketones from your fat stores, bringing about better efficiency and mental execution.

This is on the grounds that your cerebrum is the most vitality devouring organ in your body. At the point when you have a perfect and steady vitality supply from ketones, this can enable your cerebrum to work in a progressively ideal manner.

What's more, ketones are better at ensuring your mind. Studies show that ketone bodies may have cancer prevention agent properties that shield your synapses from free radicals, oxidative pressure, and harm.

In one examination performed on grown-ups with debilitated memory, the ascent of BHB ketones in their blood improved discernment.

On the off chance that you make some hard memories remaining centered, your synapses might be at fault. Your cerebrum has two fundamental synapses: glutamate and GABA.

Glutamate encourages you to structure new recollections, learn confused ideas and causes your synapses to speak with one another.

GABA is the thing that helps control glutamate. Glutamate can make your synapses overly energized. In the event that this happens, again and again, it can cause synapses to quit working and, in the end, kick the bucket. GABA is there to control and hinder glutamate. At the point when GABA levels are low, glutamate rules free, and you experience mental haze.

Ketone bodies help to forestall synapse harm by handling overabundance glutamate into GABA. Since ketones increment GABA and lessening glutamate, they help in forestalling cell harm, avoiding cell passing, and improving your psychological core interest.

As such, ketones help keep your GABA and glutamate levels adjusted, so your cerebrum remains sharp.

The effects of Intermittent Fasting on Stress Levels and Cognitive Function

Fasting has been appeared to improve memory, decrease oxidative pressure, and save learning abilities.

Researchers accept that intermittent fasting works by constraining their cells to perform better. Since your cells are under gentle pressure while fasting, the best cells adjust to this worry by improving their own capacity to adapt, while the most vulnerable cells bite the dust. This procedure is called autophagy.

This is like the pressure your body experiences when you hit the exercise center. Practicing is a type of pressure your body suffers to improve and get more grounded, as long as you rest enough after your exercises. This additionally applies to intermittent fasting, and as long as you keep on shifting back and forth between ordinary dietary patterns and fasting, it can keep on profiting you.

The entirety of this implies the keto intermittent fasting blend is ground-breaking and can help improve your intellectual capacity, on account of the defensive and stimulating impacts of ketones just as the gentle cell stress brought about by fasting.

The Keto Intermittent Fasting Connection

The ketogenic diet and intermittent fasting share huge numbers of similar health benefits in light of the fact that the two methods can have a similar outcome: a condition of ketosis.

Ketosis has numerous physical and mental benefits, from weight and fat loss to improved feelings of anxiety, mental capacity, and life span.

In any case, it's critical to remember that on the off chance that you adopt a milder strategy to intermittent keto fasting — for instance, eating inside an 8-hour window — you most likely won't enter ketosis (particularly in the event that you eat a high measure of carbs during that window).

Not every person who attempts intermittent fasting plans to enter ketosis. Indeed, on the off chance that somebody who fasts likewise eats high-carb foods, there's a generally excellent possibility they'll never enter ketosis.

Then again, if ketosis is the objective, you can utilize intermittent keto fasting as an instrument to arrive and improve your overall health.

Keto and IF Diet Plan

Possibly you're contemplating attempting the keto diet or exploring different avenues regarding fasting. Maybe you're now doing both. In any case, we've given an example every day and week by week plan of what an arrangement may resemble for somebody on a keto diet, which is additionally incorporating some other day fasting and 16:8 time-confined sustaining into their routine.

Sunday

6:00 am: Water as well as dark espresso (no, espresso won't break the fast)

9:00 am More water or dark espresso.

12:00pm: TRF closes. Have a keto-accommodating meal: possibly a serving of mixed greens with the flame-broiled chicken beat with olive oil and feta cheddar, avocado, and some hard-bubbled eggs or bacon bits.

3:00 pm: Snack on certain nuts or have some nut margarine, and possibly espresso with some MCT oil or coconut oil.

6:00 pm: 8 - 12oz of a greasy cut of meat (ribeye steak or greasy fish) in addition to certain vegetables; perhaps Brussels grows cooked in the spread.

8:00 pm: Small nibble of nuts, blueberries, and a bit of solid dull chocolate for "dessert." This is the last meal of the day.

Monday: Same eating window as yesterday: 12 - 8 pm.

Tuesday: Fasting day. No calories devoured today.

Wednesday: Eating time of 12 - 8 pm. You may be hungrier today since you fasted yesterday, particularly on the off chance that you did an early morning exercise today.

Thursday: Fasting day

Friday: 12 - 8 eating window. Exercise in the first part of the day or, in the event that you need to do an energized exercise do as such in the middle of lunch and supper.

Saturday: Fast day

Keep in mind; this is just a single model out of an about a boundless number of emphasis! Switch this up to accommodate your way of life; use it as a manual to plan your own fasting routine.

Health Benefits of Keto and Intermittent Fasting

Concentrating on the health benefits of the keto diet and fasting will assist you with remaining persuaded and to progress forward. They can include:

- Decreased levels of insulin

- Reduction in irritation (related with numerous constant illnesses)

- Weight loss

- Heart health (diminished cholesterol levels and circulatory strain)

- Autophagy – the body stalls old cells and reuses them.

- Increased vitality

- Increased center

2. Defining Specific Measurable Goals

Rather than defining an objective of getting more fit, be progressively explicit, center around basic, feasible objectives that should be possible week by week.

• Taking a walk three days per week

• Drink in any event 64 ounces of water multiple times this week

• Skip one meal this week

3. Self Reward When Reaching Mini-Goals

Set yourself up for proceeded with progress by utilizing a prize framework.

• After shedding fifteen pounds, get yourself some new garments.

• If you meet all your particular objectives referenced above for one month at that point, get a back rub.

• Have a nice decent meal for meeting week after week objectives. (It's now keto affirmed!).

The cash spared by avoiding a meal (or two) can pay for your prize! Different components spur every one of us, so make certain to make sense of what might work best for you, and you'll remain persuaded to arrive at all your objectives. Next, we should see how to begin your first fast.

Step by step instructions to Start Fasting

In this way, presently, you have the fundamentals of keto and IF and some inspiration. However, perhaps you're not feeling prepared to jump into a 16 hour fast your first day. That is no issue. The vast majority need to slide into fasting to get adjusted and gain certainty. In this way, here's a suggested procedure.

The 16:8 fast is the least demanding one to begin. It's made simpler to some degree by the way that when you get up in the first part of the day, you've just fasted for a few hours. So the entirety of that is required is to go only a couple of something else. Start by moving your morning meal up by 60 minutes. That could be one hour out of every day or week, relying upon how fastly you need to achieve your objective. At the point when you've moved your morning meal up to where it's near lunch, say 10:00 o'clock, for example, skip breakfast. Presently lunch should begin 16 hours after your supper the earlier night. So lunch would begin around early afternoon if your supper was at 8 pm. Proceed with this technique for the 24 hours and exchange day fasting.

Test Keto and Intermittent Fasting Meal Plan

Notwithstanding inspiration, realizing the guidelines with respect to what you put in your mouth is a large portion of the fight when you attempt to do keto and intermittent fasting. An example meal plan follows so as to make life somewhat simpler. Look at these basic plans.

The accompanying example plan will follow the ketogenic diet alongside 16/8 intermittent fasting. It will be ideal if you note that fasting will happen from 8 pm until noon the next day.

Monday – A glass of water and espresso before Noon. Lunch is a fish plate of mixed greens (canned fish, celery, mayo, avocado cut) and a side serving of mixed greens with farm dressing. A bite is a bunch of nuts and string cheddar. Supper is a bunless cheeseburger beat with spinach, avocado fruit, and mushrooms and a side of zucchini noodles (doodles).

Tuesday – Begin the day with a major glass of water and espresso if necessary. Bite comprises of celery and nutty spread. Supper this evening is barbecued sirloin steak bested with mushrooms, simmered broccoli, and cauliflower squash.

Wednesday – Water and espresso, not surprisingly. Breakfast is for lunch, fried eggs, avocado, and bacon are on the menu. Tidbit is a hardboiled egg and a few cucumbers. Supper is salmon cooked with lemon and dill, asparagus, and blended berries for dessert.

Thursday – Wake up to water and espresso. Lunch is a barbecued chicken plate of mixed greens with hard bubbled eggs, avocado, and sunflower seeds. Tidbit is a plate of olives, pickles, and cheddar. Supper would be cabbage and frankfurter with broccoli serving of mixed greens as a side (broccoli, mayo, bacon, almonds).

Friday – Morning water and espresso. Lunch is a sub in a tub (destroyed lettuce, tomato, pickles, olives, cheddar, ham, salami bested with olive oil and red wine vinegar). Celery sticks with cream cheddar can be included for a touch of crunch. Tidbit comprises of meat jerky and string cheddar. Supper is chicken wings and a side plate of mixed greens with farm dressing.

Saturday – Water and espresso before Noon. Lunch is eggroll in a bowl – destroyed cabbage, ground pork, and coconut aminos (fill in for soy sauce) with a side of kale chips. The bite is nuts and pepperoni. Pizza is for supper, with a cauliflower outside layer obviously, alongside a major bowl of broccoli or a side plate of mixed greens.

Sunday – The typical water and espresso. Lunch is a taco serving of mixed greens. Tidbit comprises veggies and plunge, and supper is a pot broil with green beans and cauliflower squash.

In spite of the fact that excluded, ordinary pastry can likewise be eaten after your meal. Some great decisions are blended berries, Lily's dull chocolate, or curds blended in with strawberries. In case you're searching for some keto benevolent sweet plans, look at these.

The above menu is only an example of what you can eat. When you become progressively experienced with the diet and fasting, by and large, you'll have the option to think of other innovative plans to incorporate into your meals. Keeping meals straightforward, while including assortment, will help keep you on target and keep you from getting exhausted with your food and going to unhealthy choices.

Despite the fact that you can surely nibble during the 8-hour eating window, it's a smart thought to reduce the snacks as you get more accustomed to the keto diet and (IF). Each time you eat, insulin is discharged, which turns off fat copying for 2-3 hours. In this way, refraining from nibbling will help you in your weight-loss objectives also. Next, how about we cover some average mistakes.

Basic Mistakes

The Intermittent Fasting Myths and Mistakes that Make You Gain Weight

In case You've been fasting and following the keto diet for half a month, however not getting in shape – what's the issue? It tends to be so disappointing and makes you need to surrender when you don't get results immediately, yet there might be a few reasons you're not losing the weight.

1. Such a large number of Carbs

This is presumably the number 1 suspect for those new to keto and intermittent fasting. Despite the fact that you're devouring low carb veggies, there might be shrouded sugars that are causing your weight loss to slow down. Is it true that you are devouring sugar-free items? Provided that this is true, they most likely contain sorbitol, xylitol, or some other shrouded sugar, and you might be eating a lot of them without realizing the impact it's having on you. Many sugar substitutes can cause raised insulin levels, which slows down your weight loss.

Avoid locally acquired serving of mixed greens dressings and sauces as they commonly contain a great deal of covered up carbs.

Pick keto cordial forms rather, for example, those made by Primal Kitchen. Or on the other hand, make your own keto sauces. Natively constructed mayonnaise (formula here), for example, is the reason for farm serving of mixed greens dressing. Finding the offender that is slowing down your advancement will propel you to get once more into gear.

2. You're Not in Ketosis

While you're following the diet for those initial hardly any weeks, you accept you've arrived at ketosis; however, that isn't generally the situation. Amateurs to keto and intermittent fasting are particularly vulnerable to this act of thought. Most importantly, you just might be recording and figuring your intake inaccurately. It's ideal for checking, and that should be possible through pee strips that you can purchase anyplace, from drugstores to on the web. For the best precision, get a decent blood ketone screen or ketone breath analyzer.

3. Eating Too Much

Because you're viewing your carb intake doesn't mean you can go wild with the various food gatherings. Eating a larger number of calories than you consume will, in any case, make you put on weight, keto, or not. You additionally should know that the fats you're eating have more calories, so you may need to review the sum you're devouring. Likewise, recollect that as you get thinner, the measure of calories your body needs will diminish. It is judicious to monitor that information and reevaluate your checks every ten pounds you lose. I energetically prescribe utilizing a food tracker, for example, Carb Manager to monitor your food intake.

4. An excessive amount of Protein

Here once more, you may need to recalculate your protein prerequisites. An excessive amount of protein can cause gluconeogenesis, a procedure that changes over protein into sugar. Likewise, you might need to avoid fluid protein, for example, shakes or beverages, as they may change over to sugar faster.

5. Not Fasting Long Enough

In the event that a 16:8 fast isn't delivering weight loss, go for a more extended or progressively prohibitive fast, for example, the other day fast. You can begin by doing it once per week and stir your way up to 3 times each week.

The other day fast is most likely the best fasting type for weight loss. By consolidating it with the keto diet, you'll experience substantially less appetite accordingly, making it significantly more economical also.

6. A lot of Fasting.

If fasting over 16 hours, you shouldn't take fast consecutive days. Doing as such, over time, can wreck your digestion. Substitute day fasting as of now has that admonition worked in. As indicated by Thomas DeLauer, in a different video, you have to enjoy a reprieve from fasting each third week for a time of the multi-week. This assists with resetting your digestion so you can keep profiting by your fasts.

Clearly, in case you're new to keto and intermittent fasting, this won't be an issue for some time. The significant thing to recollect is that an excess of fasting will, in the end, bring down your digestion. In this way, to avoid weight loss level on keto and intermittent fasting, don't fast consecutive days and don't fast such a large number of weeks straight.

By avoiding the above mistakes, a level on keto and intermittent fasting can be forestalled.

Moreover, probably the greatest ascribe to any fruitful way of life is arranging. Keto and intermittent fasting are the same. Finding the occasions that are directly for you to fast is basic for progress. Arranging meals and tidbits and adhering to that arrangement are basic. Most importantly, you have to know the essentials of the ketogenic diet and how intermittent fasting functions so as to discover the achievement you hunger for.

Tips for Success

Most importantly, the way that you need to attempt the keto and intermittent fasting way of life is the initial step to evolving. It shows that you need to shed pounds and improve your health. It may not generally be simple, yet here are a couple of tips to help you en route.

1. Track Your Food

There are a lot of applications that will let you track the measure of calories, carbs, and truly whatever else you need to follow. Knowing how much and what you're placing into your body can have a significant effect on progress and disappointment. Ensure the application is for the keto diet.

2. Discover a Community

Clearly, changing your way of life can be hard. Not all your loved ones may comprehend your new diet or what you're experiencing. It's imperative to have someplace you can go to talk and examine high points and low points or any inquiries. In the event that you don't have a companion or mate that is doing the diet with you at that point, don't fear, there's a lot of online networks that can help spur and bolster you in your period of scarcity.

3. Continue onward

At the point when first beginning with the keto diet and fasting, you may see the weight fall off rapidly yet then start to slow down. This is the point at which many individuals choose it's not working for them and quit. You have to recollect; it set aside some effort to put that weight on, it'll set aside some effort to fall off. It's a procedure, and you'll have to stay with it so as to see the outcomes you need. Regardless of whether you've tumbled off the wagon, you have to get dust yourself off and get directly back on.

Intermittent fasting and the Mediterranean diet

On the other side, the Mediterranean diet has been attempted and tried and is famous as perhaps the healthiest diet on the planet – with a great deal of good quality logical proof to demonstrate it. It's especially gainful for heart health, yet has additionally been appeared to build life span and secure against some incessant sicknesses.

Wealthy in plant foods like vegetables, vegetables, and whole grains (read: not the pivot of pails of pasta and gigantic sections of lasagne that a great many people wish for), it's anything but difficult to perceive any reason why this diet is so bravo. The Med diet likewise has a solid spotlight on healthy fats, to be specific additional virgin olive oil, yet additionally nuts and seafood. Furthermore, there are no limited foods. Hell, even red wine is on the menu!

Intermittent fasting and run diet

An abbreviation for Dietary Approaches to Stop Hypertension. The DASH diet is demonstrated not exclusively to diminish circulatory strain, however, help with weight loss and decrease your danger of numerous incessant infections, as well. Low in sodium yet high in potassium, calcium, and magnesium – organic product, veggies, and diminished fat dairy are the foundation of the DASH diet. Vegetables, nuts and seeds, whole grains, lean meat, and fish are incorporated too.

What's more, there you have it! Five diets that really have a few reasons to be taken seriously. Be that as it may, before you focus on either, here's my promise of caution: on the grounds that these diets could be advantageous, doesn't mean you ought to go hellfire for calfskin. As opposing as it sounds, as a dietitian, I'm not an aficionado of 'diets.' That is on the grounds that they lead to the unavoidable dieting cycle, in which you're bound by a lot of rules and afterward feel regretful once you in the long run 'slip up.'

In the event that weight loss is your objective, instead of beginning another 'diet' that is going to overhaul your whole method for eating, I'd urge you to concentrate on little, practical changes you can adhere to, for good. Take your pick of components of each diet recorded over that will suit you, and work towards them, progressively. That way, you'll develop a collection of healthy propensities over time, and be obviously better off eventually.

Plant-Based Intermittent Fasting for Vegans

The vegan fasting variant of this weight loss technique can accompany splendid intermittent fasting results, in spite of the fact that it could, in any case, be a troublesome procedure for even the most committed of vegans.

If you have been focusing on anything on the planet over the most recent quite a long while, there is a decent possibility that you have at any rate known about something that is called intermittent fasting. The intermittent fasting diet comes in a few different structures, some of which incorporate doing a 5:2 diet, 16:8 diet, just as a few different varieties also.

Indeed, the thing about intermittent fasting is that it works. This implies it has become the most up to date weight loss rage and has been developing in its notoriety faster than some other diet before it. Also, to make sure you realize this is a genuine article, next time you head outside, simply search for the individual stepping around the local who hasn't eaten over the most recent 14 hours and is perceptibly 'hangry.'

Beneath we go over the essential strides to beginning intermittent vegan fasting:

1. Create a feasible guide: Take a gander at your life, your work hours, and your propensities. Do you will, in general, tidbit around lunch? Do you skip breakfast a great deal? Would you be able to abandon food for quite a while, or do you get bad-tempered rapidly?

For the vast majority, the 16:8 diet is the most effortless diet to adhere to, eating around the hours of 11 am – 7 pm.

2. Adopt it gradually: There's no compelling reason to "bounce in at the profound end" and make your body believe it's out of nowhere going to starve to death. On the off chance that it works better for you, take a stab at the beginning with a 10-hour or 12-hour eating window before dropping down to the 8-hour window. Likewise, in case you're making the 5:2 arrangement, attempt it as a 6:1 diet from the start.

3.Set an audit date: Set an end date for your fasting, regardless of whether it's two weeks or 2 months from now. If you haven't gotten the outcomes you were seeking after by, at that point, maybe intermittent fasting isn't the correct eating plan for you.

4. Plan your food: Okay, the general purpose of fasting is that you shouldn't meal plan excessively. In any case, in case you're eating a crude vegan or plant-based diet, you have to search out supplements and fiber-filled meals, which will limit your craving and hunger during any fast periods.

Who Should Try Vegan Intermittent Fasting

1. Vegans who need to get thinner and get conditioned: Fast vegan weight loss is, in fact, conceivable with fasting, making it simpler for you to shed pounds and get the body you want.

2. Vegans who need to improve their exhibition at the exercise center: Studies propose that intermittent fasting supports development hormones by as much as 600%, making vegan increases simpler than any time in recent memory in the rec center.

3. Vegans who need to grow better dietary patterns: Some vegans eat unhealthy food absentmindedly. Plant-based intermittent fasting constrains you to create healthier dietary patterns.

Who Should Not Try Intermittent Fasting

1. Vegans who are pregnant or breastfeeding: If you're a vegan who is pregnant or breastfeeding, try not to explore different avenues regarding diets and fasting methods. Your infant is developing and is depending on you for a consistent progression of supplements.

2. Vegans who are diabetic: Although a few sources guarantee that fasting could help with diabetes, it is by and large prescribed that diabetics ought not fast, as the procedure could upset their glucose levels.

IMPORTANCE OF LIFESTYLE

Intermittent fasting has been appeared to diminish irritation in your body.

In any case, liquor may advance aggravation, checking the impacts of this diet.

Ceaseless aggravation may advance different ailments, for example, heart ailment, type 2 diabetes, and certain malignancies.

Research shows that the irritation from extreme drinking may prompt broken gut disorder, bacterial overgrowth, and a lopsidedness in gut microscopic organisms.

High liquor intake can likewise overwhelm your liver, diminishing its capacity to sift through possibly destructive poisons.

Together, these consequences for your gut and liver may advance aggravation all through your body, which over time, can prompt organ harm.

Over the top liquor, intake can cause far-reaching aggravation in your body, checking the impacts of intermittent fasting and conceivably prompting infections.

Drinking liquor can break your fast

During a fast, you should avoid all foods and refreshments for a set measure of time.

In particular, intermittent fasting is intended to advance hormonal and substance changes —, for example, fat consuming and cell fix — that may profit your health.

As liquor contains calories, any measure of it during a fasting period will break your fast.

No different, it is flawlessly worthy of drinking with some restraint during your eating periods.

Liquor may forestall cell fix.

During fasting periods, your body starts cell fix forms like autophagy, in which old, harmed proteins are expelled from cells to produce more up to date, healthier cells.

This procedure may diminish your danger of malignancy, advance enemy of maturing impacts, and at any rate somewhat clarify why calorie limitation has been appeared to expand life expectancy.

Ongoing creature contemplates showing that ceaseless liquor intake may hinder autophagy in the liver and fat tissue. Remember that human examinations are required

As liquor contains calories, drinking any sum during a fasting period will break you're fast and may forestall cell fix forms.

Picking better liquor choices

As liquor breaks your fast whenever expended during a fasting period, it's prescribed to just drink during your assigned eating periods. You ought to likewise hold your intake under tight restraints. Moderate liquor consumption is characterized as close to 1 beverage for every day for women and close to 2 every day for men.

While intermittent fasting doesn't have exacting standards for food and drink intake, some liquor decisions are healthier than others and more averse to check your dietary routine.

Healthier choices incorporate dry wine and hard spirits, as they're lower in calories. You can taste these all alone or blended in with soft drink water.

To constrain your sugar and calorie intake, avoid blended beverages, and better wines.

During intermittent fasting, it's ideal for savoring liquor moderate sums and just during your eating periods. Healthier choices incorporate dry wine and hard spirits.

Unhindered Eating

Any individual who has ever changed their diet to accomplish a health advantage or arrive at a healthy weight realizes that you begin to desire foods that you are advised not to eat. Truth be told, an investigation distributed in 2017 affirmed that an expanded drive to eat is a key factor during a weight loss journey.4

Be that as it may, this test is explicitly constrained on an intermittent fasting plan. Food limitation just happens during certain constrained hours, and on the non-fasting hours or days of the arrangement, you can, for the most part, eat anything you desire. Truth be told, specialists here and there call nowadays "devouring" days.

Obviously, proceeding to eat unhealthy foods may not be the healthiest method to pick up benefits from intermittent fasting; however, removing them during specific days constrains your overall intake and may at last give benefits.

Might Boost Longevity

One of the most broadly referred to benefits of intermittent fasting includes life span. As indicated by the

So does this advantage stretch out to people? As indicated by the individuals who advance the diets, it does. Be that as it may, long haul examines are expected to affirm the advantage. As indicated by an audit distributed in 2010, there has been observational research connecting strict fasting too long haul life span benefits, yet it was difficult to decide whether fasting gave the advantage or whenever related components played a part.5

Advances Weight Loss

In an audit of intermittent fasting research distributed in 2018, creators report that the examinations they inspected demonstrated a noteworthy reduction in fat mass among subjects who took an interest in clinical preliminaries. They additionally saw that intermittent fasting was found as productive in decreasing weight, independent of the body mass index.6

It is conceivable, nonetheless, that IF is not anymore viable than conventional calorie limitation.

RACKING NAD JOURNALLING

Food Diary - How to keep the track of What You Eat

Recording what you eat resembles seeing a day of food spread out before you.

You can recognize your great propensities, (for example, eating three everyday meals and picking healthy bites) and your unfortunate propensities, (for example, unhealthy nibbling late around evening time and drinking for the most part sugary beverages).

There is a varieties of approaches to monitor what you eat. You can record it on paper, keep notes on your PC or advanced gadget, or utilize a diet following site or application. You track the occasions you eat, the foods you eat, partition sizes, and notes about what you were doing or feeling at the time utilizing a large portion of these methods.

By the day's end, audit your food list (Food Diary) and pose these inquiries:

To control hunger:

- Did I eat healthy meals?

- Did I have filling foods (counting water) with each meal or each bite?

- Did I eat enough natural products, vegetables, and fiber from entire grains?

- Did I plan for healthy eating to help overcome yearnings?

To decrease calories:

- Did I keep parcels little?

- Did I limit sugary, unhealthy foods, and drinks?

- Did I incorporate foods grown from the ground with each meal or tidbit?

- Did I eat when I was not ravenous? On the off chance that indeed, what was I feeling or doing that caused me to eat?

THE 7-DAYS INTERMITTENT FASTING MEAL PLAN FOR FAST RESULTS

In case you don't know what to eat on the intermittent fasting meal plan, we've assembled a 7-day meal intend to kick your off on the correct foot! The plans are perfect and healthy, yet additionally extraordinarily tasty so you can appreciate them while viewing your waistline. Whether of which strategy you pick, we have you covered with this fledgling 7-day eating plan!

16/8 Intermittent Fasting Meal Plan

Monday

- Meal #1: Avocado chicken plate of mixed greens

- Snack #2: Hand loaded with nuts

- Meal #3: Keto Spicy Chicken Sauté Tossed With Avocado

Tuesday

- Meal #1: Taco lettuce wraps

- Snack #2: Fruit of your decision

- Meal #3: Chicken plate of mixed greens

Wednesday

- Meal #1: Tuna avocado plate of mixed greens wrap

- Snack #2: Hummus and crude veggie sticks

- Meal #3: Asian Wings

Thursday

- Meal #1: Broccoli tofu plate of mixed greens

- Snack #2: Piece of dull chocolate

- Meal #3: Salmon kale plate of mixed greens

Friday

- Meal #1: Turkey Chili

- Snack #2: Almonds

- Meal #3: Grilled chicken plate of mixed greens

Saturday

- Meal #1: Grilled salmon plate of mixed greens

- Snack #2: Dark chocolate bark

- Meal #3: Chicken tortilla soup

Sunday

- Meal #1: Sprouts, chicken, quinoa Buddha bowl

- Snack #2: Greek yogurt

- Meal #3: Teriyaki chicken with cauliflower rice

Intermittent fasting doesn't need to be a frightening thing. When can you eat these flavorful meals, who wouldn't cherish this straightforward method to shed pounds?

CPSIA information can be obtained
at www.ICGtesting.com
Printed in the USA
LVHW060619260421
685568LV00009B/795